LILA HAYES

The Ultimate Low Histamine Cookbook for Beginners

Delicious Recipes for Histamine Intolerance and Mast Cell Activation Syndrome, Including a 4 Phase Histamine Reset Plan

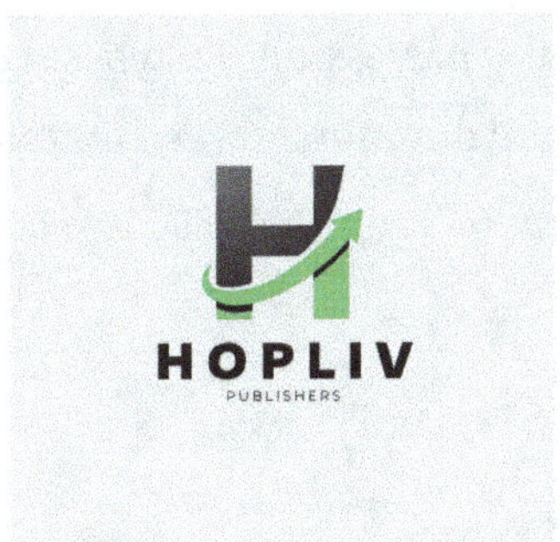

This book was professionally typeset on Reedsy.
Find out more at reedsy.com

Contents

Acknowledgement

Creating this cookbook has been a labor of love, and I am deeply grateful to everyone who has supported me along the way.

First and foremost, I would like to thank my family and friends for their unwavering support and encouragement. Your belief in me has been a constant source of motivation and inspiration.

A heartfelt thank you to all the healthcare professionals and dietitians who have shared their knowledge and expertise on histamine intolerance. Your guidance has been invaluable in shaping the content of this book.

To the members of the online histamine intolerance communities and support groups, thank you for sharing your experiences, recipes, and tips. Your insights have enriched this cookbook and made it more comprehensive and practical.

Special thanks to my recipe testers, who spent countless hours in the kitchen to ensure these recipes are both delicious and effective in managing histamine levels. Your feedback has been instrumental in perfecting each dish.

Lastly, I would like to express my gratitude to my readers. Your journey towards better health and well-being is why this book was created. Thank you for allowing me to be a part of it.

With gratitude, Lila Hayes

Introduction

Welcome to "The Ultimate Low Histamine Cookbook for Beginners: Delicious Recipes for Histamine Intolerance and Mast Cell Activation Syndrome, Including a 4 Phase Histamine Reset Plan"! If you're here, you're probably looking for ways to manage histamine intolerance without sacrificing taste or breaking the bank. Let's start by understanding what histamine intolerance is. Histamine is a natural compound found in many foods and is also produced by our bodies. It plays various roles, including helping with digestion and immune responses. However, some people have trouble breaking down histamine, leading to a build-up in the body and causing symptoms like headaches, hives, digestive issues, and more. This is what's known as histamine intolerance.

Managing histamine intolerance can be challenging, but one of the most effective ways is through diet. A low histamine diet helps to reduce the intake of histamine-rich foods, allowing your body to better manage and process the histamine it encounters. This can lead to fewer symptoms and an overall better quality of life. Eating low histamine foods doesn't mean you have to eat bland or boring meals. With the right recipes and ingredients, you can enjoy flavorful, satisfying meals while keeping your histamine levels in check.

This cookbook is designed with beginners in mind. If you're new to the world of histamine intolerance or just starting to explore a low histamine diet, you're in the right place. Each recipe is carefully crafted to be simple, easy to follow, and delicious. We understand that starting a new diet can be overwhelming, so we've included helpful tips, explanations, and guidance throughout the book. Our goal is to make your transition to a low histamine lifestyle as smooth and enjoyable as possible.

Eating healthy shouldn't have to be expensive. We know that managing a special diet can sometimes strain your budget, which is why we've focused on using affordable, easily accessible ingredients. You won't find any obscure or costly items here. Instead, we prioritize fresh, wholesome foods that you can find at your local grocery store. Additionally, the recipes are designed to be straightforward and quick, so you won't spend hours in the kitchen or need fancy equipment. This way, you can enjoy delicious, low histamine meals without stress or hassle.

We're excited to embark on this journey with you. Whether you're cooking for yourself, your family, or friends, these recipes will help you create tasty, healthy meals that everyone can enjoy. Let's get started on your path to better health and delicious eating!

Understanding Histamine Intolerance

What is Histamine?

Histamine is a naturally occurring compound found in many living organisms, including humans. It's a type of biogenic amine, which means it's a molecule derived from amino acids. Histamine plays several important roles in the body, particularly in the immune system, digestive system, and central nervous system.

Roles and Functions of Histamine:

1. **Immune Response**:

- **Allergic Reactions**: Histamine is best known for its role in allergic reactions. When your body detects an allergen (such as pollen, pet dander, or certain foods), your immune system triggers the release of histamine from mast cells and basophils. This release leads to symptoms like itching, swelling, redness, and mucus production as part of the body's effort to expel the allergen.
- **Inflammation**: Histamine helps to widen blood vessels and increase blood flow to affected areas during an immune response, contributing to inflammation and helping the body fight off infections.

1. **Digestive System**:

- **Stomach Acid Regulation**: In the stomach, histamine stimulates the production of gastric acid by binding to H2 receptors on the stomach lining. This acid is crucial for breaking down food and absorbing nutrients.

1. **Central Nervous System**:

- **Neurotransmitter**: Histamine acts as a neurotransmitter in the brain, influencing various functions such as sleep-wake cycles, appetite regulation, and cognitive processes.

Histamine in Foods:

Histamine is present in varying amounts in many foods. Some foods naturally contain high levels of histamine, while others can cause the body to release histamine or block the enzymes that break down histamine. Here are some examples:

High Histamine Foods:

- Aged cheeses
- Fermented foods (sauerkraut, kimchi, soy sauce)
- Processed meats (salami, pepperoni)
- Alcoholic beverages (especially red wine and beer)
- Certain fish (tuna, mackerel, sardines)

Histamine-Releasing Foods:

- Strawberries
- Tomatoes
- Eggplant
- Spinach
- Citrus fruits

Symptoms of Histamine Intolerance

Histamine intolerance occurs when the body accumulates too much histamine or struggles to break it down effectively. This can lead to a wide range of symptoms that often resemble allergic reactions. Because histamine affects various systems in the body, the symptoms can be diverse and sometimes confusing. Here are some common symptoms associated with histamine intolerance:

1. **Headaches and Migraines**

- Persistent or recurrent headaches
- Severe, throbbing migraines

2. **Skin Reactions**

- Hives (urticaria)
- Itching and redness
- Flushing of the face and neck
- Eczema or worsening of existing skin conditions

3. **Digestive Issues**

- Bloating and gas
- Abdominal pain and cramps
- Diarrhea or loose stools
- Nausea and vomiting

4. **Respiratory Symptoms**

- Nasal congestion and sinus problems
- Runny nose and sneezing
- Difficulty breathing or shortness of breath
- Asthma-like symptoms

5. Cardiovascular Symptoms

- Rapid or irregular heartbeat (tachycardia)
- Low blood pressure (hypotension)
- Dizziness or lightheadedness
- Fluctuations in blood pressure

6. Neurological Symptoms

- Fatigue and lethargy
- Anxiety or panic attacks
- Irritability and mood swings
- Difficulty concentrating or brain fog

7. Eye Symptoms

- Watery, red, or itchy eyes
- Swelling around the eyes (periorbital edema)

8. Other Symptoms

- Swelling of tissues (angioedema), particularly in the face, lips, and throat
- Menstrual irregularities in women
- Sensitivity to certain foods or alcohol
- Increased sensitivity to environmental allergens

Why These Symptoms Occur

Histamine is a compound involved in immune responses, digestion, and neurotransmission. When histamine levels become too high or when the body cannot break it down efficiently, it can bind to receptors in various tissues and organs, causing the symptoms listed above. The severity and combination of symptoms can vary greatly from person to person, making histamine intolerance a challenging condition to diagnose.

Managing Symptoms

The key to managing histamine intolerance is to reduce histamine intake through dietary changes and possibly using supplements to support histamine breakdown. Identifying and avoiding high-histamine foods and other triggers can significantly alleviate symptoms. Additionally, consulting with a health-care professional who understands histamine intolerance can provide further guidance and support.

Understanding these symptoms can help you recognize and manage histamine intolerance more effectively. By making informed dietary choices and adopting a low histamine lifestyle, many people find significant relief from their symptoms and enjoy a better quality of life.

Foods High in Histamine

Managing histamine intolerance often starts with understanding which foods are high in histamine and may trigger symptoms. Here are some common high-histamine foods:

1. **Fermented Foods and Beverages**

- Sauerkraut
- Kimchi
- Soy sauce
- Vinegar and vinegar-containing foods (like pickles and mustard)
- Alcoholic beverages (especially wine, beer, and champagne)

2. **Aged and Processed Meats**

- Salami
- Pepperoni

- Ham
- Sausages
- Smoked meats and fish

3. **Aged Cheeses**

- Cheddar
- Gouda
- Parmesan
- Blue cheese
- Swiss

4. **Certain Fish**

- Tuna
- Mackerel
- Sardines
- Anchovies
- Herring

5. **Other High-Histamine Foods**

- Tomatoes
- Eggplant
- Spinach
- Avocado
- Certain nuts (like walnuts and cashews)

Foods Low in Histamine

On the other hand, many foods are low in histamine and generally safer for those with histamine intolerance. Here are some examples:

1. **Fresh Meats and Poultry**

• Freshly cooked beef, chicken, turkey, and lamb (avoid aged or processed)

2. **Fresh Fish**

- Cod
- Haddock
- Sole
- Freshly cooked fish (not canned or smoked)

3. **Fruits**

- Apples
- Pears
- Blueberries
- Cherries
- Watermelon

4. **Vegetables**

- Carrots
- Zucchini
- Broccoli
- Kale
- Lettuce

5. **Grains and Legumes**

- Rice
- Quinoa
- Oats
- Lentils
- Chickpeas

6. **Dairy Alternatives**

- Rice milk
- Coconut milk
- Almond milk (if tolerated)

Tips for Managing Histamine Levels

Managing histamine intolerance effectively involves more than just choosing the right foods. Here are some practical tips to help you keep your histamine levels in check:

1. **Eat Fresh and Cook from Scratch**:

- Fresh foods typically have lower histamine levels. Prepare meals at home using fresh ingredients to avoid preservatives and additives that can increase histamine levels.

1. **Avoid Leftovers**:

- Histamine levels in food can increase over time. Try to eat meals soon after preparing them and avoid keeping leftovers for more than a day.

1. **Freeze Extra Portions**:

- If you need to prepare food in advance, freeze portions immediately after cooking. This helps prevent histamine from forming as the food sits in the refrigerator.

1. **Be Cautious with Fermented and Aged Foods**:

- Limit or avoid fermented, aged, and processed foods, as they tend to be high in histamine.

1. **Stay Hydrated**:

- Drink plenty of water throughout the day. Staying hydrated can help your body process histamine more effectively.

1. **Try Low-Histamine Substitutes**:

- Use low-histamine alternatives for common high-histamine ingredients. For example, use fresh herbs instead of aged cheeses for flavor, or coconut aminos instead of soy sauce.

1. **Monitor and Rotate Foods**:

- Keep a food diary to track what you eat and how it affects your symptoms. Rotating foods every few days can also help prevent a build-up of histamine.

1. **Consult with a Healthcare Professional**:

- Work with a dietitian or healthcare provider familiar with histamine intolerance to create a personalized plan that meets your nutritional needs while managing histamine levels.

By following these tips and choosing low-histamine foods, you can better manage histamine intolerance and enjoy a varied and satisfying diet.

Kitchen Essentials

Basic Kitchen Tools and Equipment

Having the right tools in your kitchen can make preparing low histamine meals easier and more enjoyable. Here's a list of basic kitchen tools and equipment that will help you get started:

1. **Cutting Board and Knives**

- A durable cutting board (preferably non-porous like plastic or bamboo)
- A sharp chef's knife
- A paring knife for smaller tasks

2. **Measuring Tools**

- Measuring cups for both dry and liquid ingredients
- Measuring spoons

3. **Mixing Bowls**

- A set of mixing bowls in various sizes

4. **Pots and Pans**

- A large and medium saucepan

- A large skillet or frying pan
- A stockpot for soups and stews

5. Baking Sheets and Casserole Dishes

- Baking sheets for roasting vegetables and baking
- Casserole dishes for oven meals

6. Cooking Utensils

- Wooden spoons for stirring
- Spatulas for flipping and mixing
- Tongs for handling hot food

7. Appliances

- A blender for smoothies and purees
- A food processor for chopping and mixing
- A slow cooker or Instant Pot for easy, hands-off cooking

8. Storage Containers

- Airtight containers for storing leftovers and prepped ingredients
- Freezer bags for freezing portions

9. Other Essentials

- A colander for draining pasta and washing vegetables
- A grater for zesting and shredding
- A whisk for mixing

Essential Low Histamine Pantry Staples

Stocking your pantry with low histamine staples ensures you always have the ingredients you need to prepare healthy and delicious meals. Here are some key items to include:

1. **Grains and Legumes**

- White and brown rice
- Quinoa
- Oats
- Lentils
- Chickpeas (dried or canned)

2. **Flours and Baking Supplies**

- Rice flour
- Coconut flour
- Gluten-free flour blend
- Baking powder (ensure it's low histamine)
- Arrowroot powder or cornstarch for thickening

3. **Pasta and Noodles**

- Rice noodles
- Gluten-free pasta
- Quinoa pasta

4. **Oils and Fats**

- Olive oil
- Coconut oil
- Avocado oil

5. Canned Goods (Low Histamine)

- Coconut milk
- Low sodium chicken or vegetable broth (ensure it's low histamine)
- Plain, unsweetened applesauce

6. Nuts and Seeds

- Almonds (if tolerated)
- Pumpkin seeds
- Sunflower seeds

7. Sweeteners

- Honey (if tolerated)
- Maple syrup
- Coconut sugar

8. Herbs and Spices

- Fresh or dried herbs (basil, oregano, thyme, rosemary)
- Ground turmeric
- Ground ginger
- Garlic powder (if tolerated)

9. Condiments and Sauces

- Coconut aminos (a low histamine soy sauce alternative)
- Homemade mayo (using fresh ingredients)
- Unsweetened coconut yogurt

10. Beverages

- Herbal teas (chamomile, rooibos, peppermint)
- Coconut water
- Freshly squeezed fruit juices

Tips for Stocking Your Low Histamine Pantry

1. **Buy Fresh When Possible**: Opt for fresh, unprocessed ingredients whenever you can. Fresh foods generally have lower histamine levels.
2. **Check Labels**: Always read labels to ensure there are no hidden high-histamine ingredients or additives.
3. **Rotate Stock**: Keep your pantry organized and use the oldest items first to ensure nothing goes to waste.
4. **Bulk Buying**: Purchase staple items in bulk to save money, but make sure to store them properly to prevent spoilage.
5. **Experiment with Flavors**: Don't be afraid to try new herbs and spices to keep your meals exciting and flavorful.

By equipping your kitchen with the right tools and stocking your pantry with essential low histamine staples, you'll be well-prepared to create delicious, healthy meals that fit your dietary needs.

Budget-Friendly Shopping Tips

Eating a low histamine diet doesn't have to be expensive. Here are some practical tips to help you manage your grocery budget while sticking to your dietary needs:

1. **Plan Your Meals**

- Create a weekly meal plan to avoid impulse buys and ensure you use up all your groceries.
- Make a shopping list based on your meal plan to stay focused and avoid unnecessary purchases.

2. **Buy in Bulk**

- Purchase staples like rice, oats, lentils, and beans in bulk to save money.
- Store bulk items in airtight containers to keep them fresh for longer.

3. **Shop Seasonal and Local**

- Choose fruits and vegetables that are in season for better prices and fresher produce.
- Visit local farmers' markets for good deals on fresh, low histamine foods.

4. **Use Coupons and Sales**

- Take advantage of coupons, discounts, and sales to stock up on pantry staples and fresh produce.
- Sign up for store loyalty programs to receive additional discounts and special offers.

5. **Opt for Store Brands**

- Store brands often offer the same quality as name brands but at a lower cost.
- Compare prices and ingredients to find the best deals.

6. **Minimize Processed Foods**

- Processed foods are often more expensive and can be high in histamine.
- Focus on whole, unprocessed foods to save money and improve your diet.

7. **Batch Cooking and Freezing**

- Prepare large batches of meals and freeze portions for later. This saves time and reduces food waste.

- Invest in quality freezer bags or containers to store prepped meals.

8. **Grow Your Own Herbs**

- Growing your own herbs like basil, oregano, and rosemary can save money and provide fresh flavors for your meals.
- Even a small windowsill herb garden can be a cost-effective solution.

Food Storage and Preparation Tips

Proper storage and preparation of low histamine foods can help maintain their quality and reduce histamine levels. Here are some tips to help you get the most out of your groceries:

1. **Store Foods Properly**

- Keep fresh produce in the refrigerator to slow down the production of histamine.
- Use airtight containers for storing bulk items like grains, legumes, and flours.

2. **Freeze Fresh Foods**

- Freeze fresh meats and fish as soon as you bring them home to prevent histamine build-up.
- Portion and freeze cooked meals to have low histamine options ready to go.

3. **Avoid Leftovers**

- Cook only what you need for each meal to avoid having leftovers, which can increase in histamine over time.
- If you do have leftovers, eat them within 24 hours or freeze them immediately.

4. Quick Cooling

- Cool cooked foods quickly by spreading them out in shallow containers before refrigerating or freezing.
- Avoid letting food sit out at room temperature for extended periods.

5. Choose Fresh Over Canned or Processed

- Fresh foods typically contain lower levels of histamine compared to canned or processed alternatives.
- Avoid pre-packaged and processed foods whenever possible.

6. Simple Cooking Methods

- Use simple cooking methods like steaming, baking, grilling, and boiling to preserve the nutritional value and keep histamine levels low.
- Avoid slow cooking methods for long periods, as this can increase histamine levels in some foods.

7. Use Acidic Marinades

- Acidic marinades made with lemon juice or vinegar can help reduce histamine levels in meats and fish.
- Marinate foods in the refrigerator and cook them promptly.

8. Keep a Clean Kitchen

- Maintain a clean and organized kitchen to prevent cross-contamination and food spoilage.
- Regularly clean your refrigerator, pantry, and food storage containers.

By following these budget-friendly shopping and food storage tips, you can effectively manage your histamine intolerance while keeping your grocery expenses under control. This will help you enjoy a healthy, varied diet without unnecessary stress or financial strain.

Breakfast Recipes

Berry Banana Smoothie

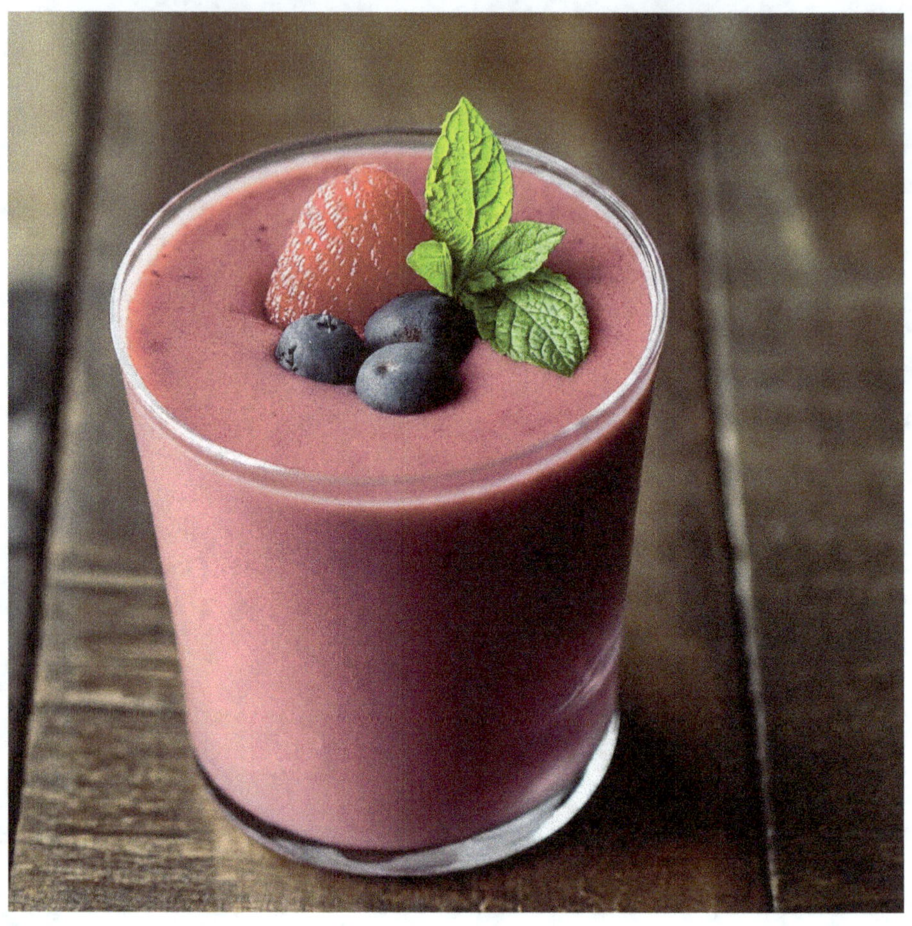

This Berry Banana Smoothie is a refreshing and nutrient-packed way to start your day. It's loaded with antioxidants, vitamins, and fiber, making it a perfect breakfast option.

Cooking Time: 5 minutes

Servings: 2

Ingredients:

- 1 cup fresh or frozen mixed berries (blueberries, strawberries, raspberries)
- 1 ripe banana
- 1 cup unsweetened almond milk (or any low-histamine milk alternative)
- 1 tablespoon chia seeds

- 1 teaspoon honey (optional, if tolerated)
- Ice cubes (optional, for a thicker smoothie)

Instructions:

1. Add the mixed berries, banana, almond milk, chia seeds, and honey to a blender.
2. Blend on high until smooth and creamy.
3. Add ice cubes if desired and blend again.
4. Pour into two glasses and serve immediately.

Tips:

- Use fresh berries to minimize histamine levels.
- You can substitute the almond milk with coconut milk or rice milk.
- Add a handful of spinach for an extra nutrient boost without altering the flavor.

Nutritional Info (per serving):

- Calories: 150
- Protein: 3g
- Carbohydrates: 35g
- Fat: 3g
- Fiber: 7g

* * *

Green Detox Juice

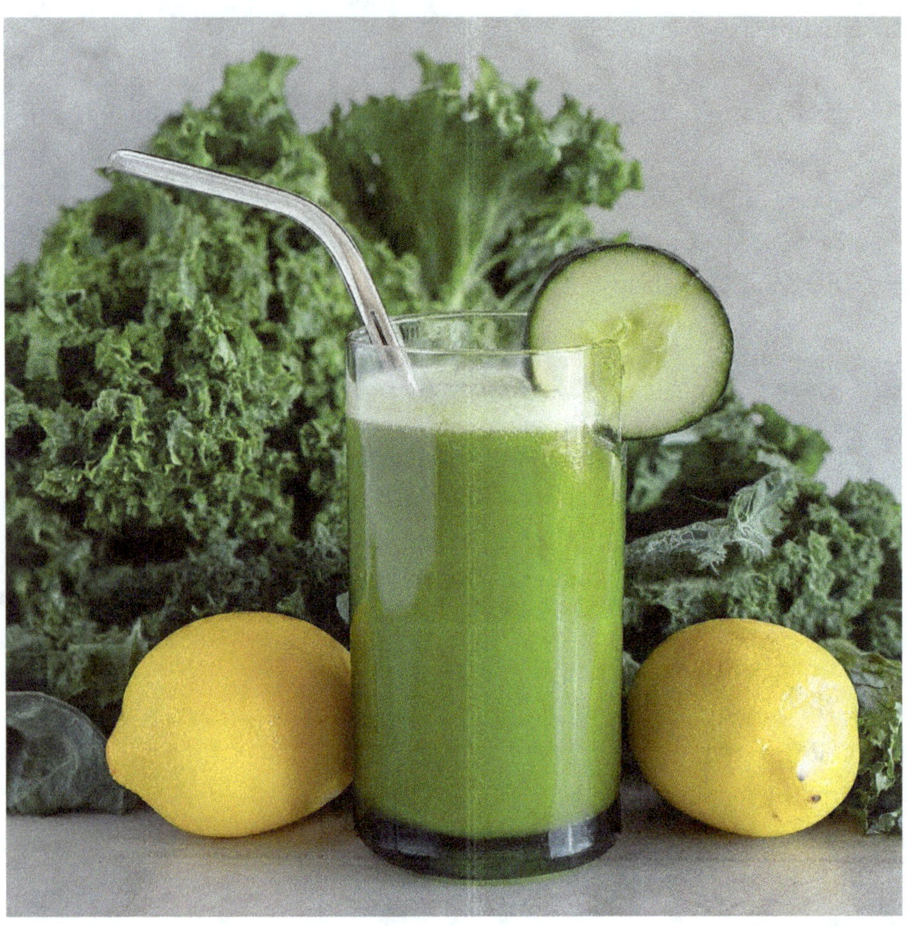

This Green Detox Juice is a fantastic way to kickstart your day with a boost of vitamins and minerals. It's refreshing, hydrating, and perfect for supporting your body's natural detox processes.

Cooking Time: 10 minutes

Servings: 2

Ingredients:

- 1 cucumber, peeled and chopped
- 2 celery stalks, chopped
- 1 green apple, cored and chopped
- 1 cup spinach leaves
- 1/2 lemon, juiced
- 1-inch piece of fresh ginger, peeled
- 1 cup cold water

Instructions:

1. Add the cucumber, celery, green apple, spinach, lemon juice, ginger, and water to a blender.
2. Blend on high until smooth.
3. Pour the mixture through a fine mesh strainer or nut milk bag into a bowl to remove the pulp.
4. Transfer the juice into glasses and serve immediately.

Tips:

- Drink the juice right after making it to maximize nutrient intake.
- Adjust the amount of ginger to your taste preference.
- Add a few ice cubes if you prefer your juice chilled.

Nutritional Info (per serving):

- Calories: 80
- Protein: 2g
- Carbohydrates: 18g
- Fat: 0g
- Fiber: 4g

* * *

Quinoa Breakfast Bowl with Fresh Berries

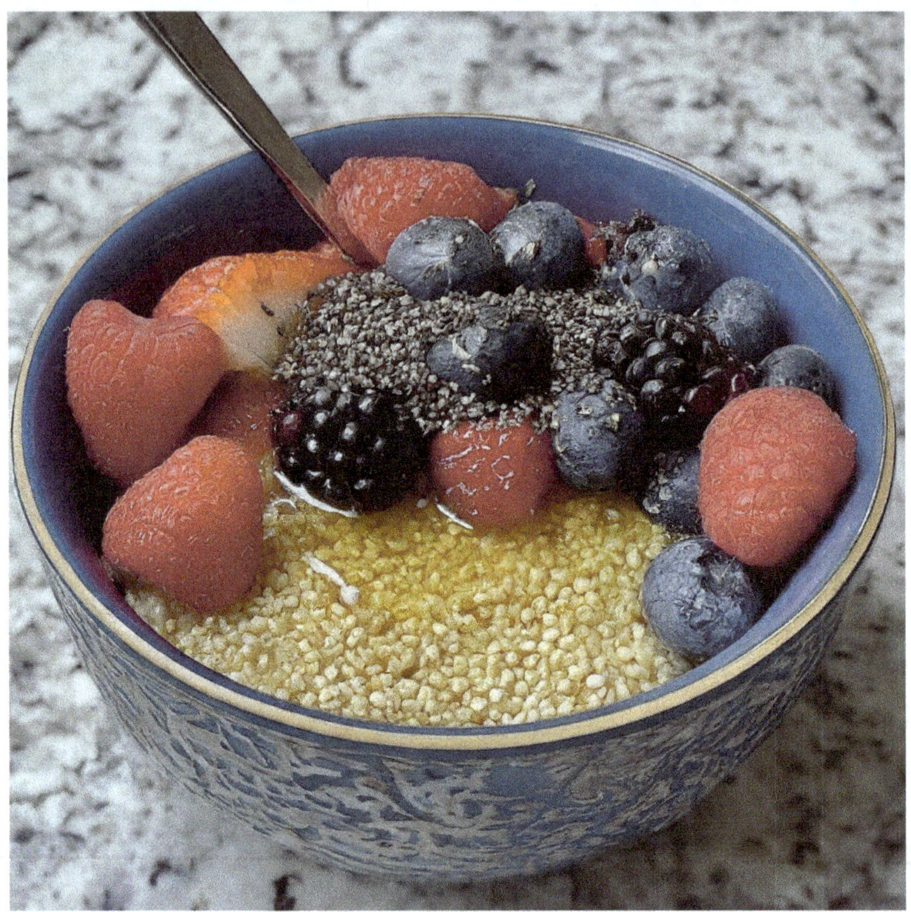

This Quinoa Breakfast Bowl with Fresh Berries is a wholesome and delicious way to start your morning. Packed with protein, fiber, and antioxidants, it's both satisfying and nutritious.

Cooking Time: 20 minutes

Servings: 2

Ingredients:

- 1 cup cooked quinoa (follow package instructions for cooking)
- 1/2 cup fresh blueberries
- 1/2 cup fresh strawberries, sliced
- 1/2 cup unsweetened almond milk (or any low-histamine milk alternative)
- 1 tablespoon chia seeds
- 1 tablespoon honey (optional, if tolerated)

Instructions:

1. Divide the cooked quinoa between two bowls.
2. Top each bowl with blueberries, strawberries, and chia seeds.
3. Drizzle with almond milk and honey if using.
4. Stir gently to combine and enjoy immediately.

Tips:

- Cook quinoa in advance and store it in the fridge for up to 3 days.
- Substitute or add other low-histamine fruits like pears or apples.
- For added crunch, sprinkle with a few pumpkin seeds or sunflower seeds.

Nutritional Info (per serving):

- Calories: 280
- Protein: 8g
- Carbohydrates: 48g
- Fat: 6g
- Fiber: 9g

* * *

Overnight Oats with Coconut Milk

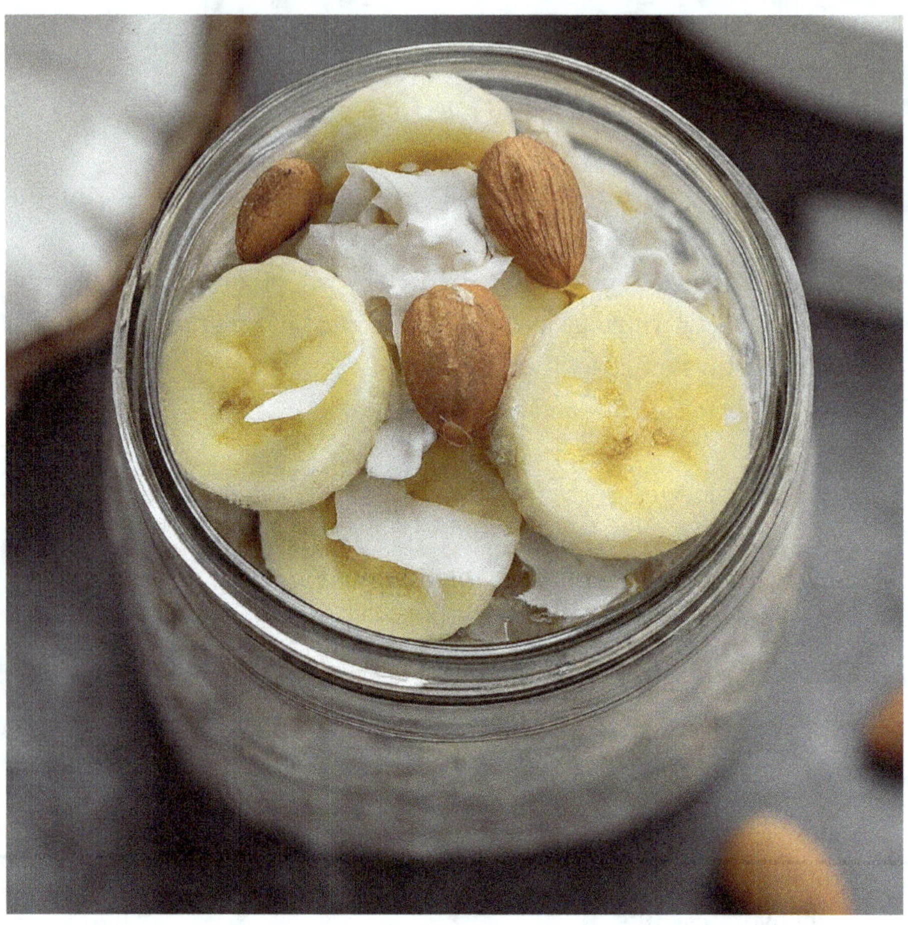

These Overnight Oats with Coconut Milk are a convenient and delicious breakfast option. Prepare them the night before for a quick, grab-and-go meal that's creamy and satisfying.

Cooking Time: 5 minutes (plus overnight soaking)

Servings: 2

Ingredients:

- 1 cup rolled oats (gluten-free if needed)
- 1 cup unsweetened coconut milk
- 1/2 cup fresh blueberries
- 1/2 cup fresh raspberries
- 1 tablespoon chia seeds
- 1 teaspoon vanilla extract
- 1 tablespoon honey (optional, if tolerated)

Instructions:

1. In a medium bowl, combine the oats, coconut milk, chia seeds, and vanilla extract.
2. Stir well to ensure the oats and chia seeds are fully incorporated with the coconut milk.
3. Divide the mixture between two jars or bowls.
4. Top each with blueberries and raspberries.
5. Cover and refrigerate overnight.
6. In the morning, drizzle with honey if using and enjoy cold or at room temperature.

Tips:

- Feel free to mix in other low-histamine fruits or nuts to customize your oats.
- If you prefer a warm breakfast, heat the oats in the microwave for 1-2 minutes before eating.
- Add a tablespoon of nut butter for extra protein and flavor.

Nutritional Info (per serving):

- Calories: 300
- Protein: 6g
- Carbohydrates: 50g

- Fat: 10g
- Fiber: 10g

* * *

Avocado Toast with Fresh Herbs

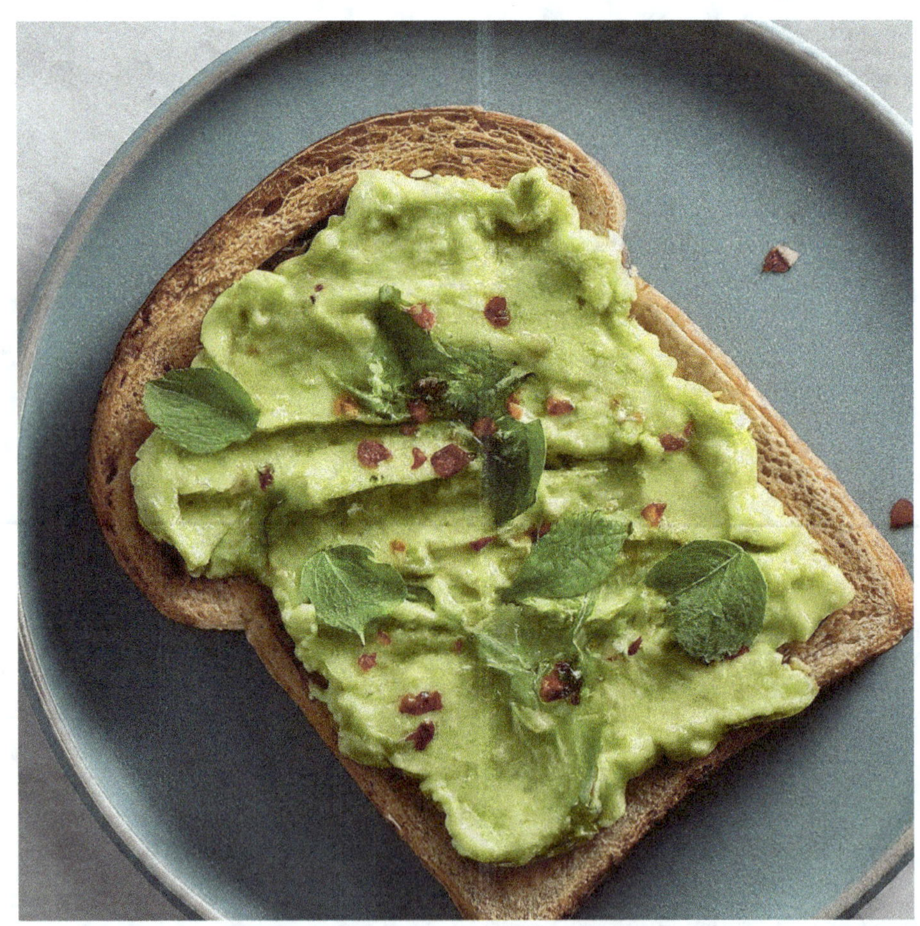

Avocado Toast with Fresh Herbs is a simple yet flavorful breakfast option. It's packed with healthy fats, fiber, and a burst of freshness from the herbs, making it a perfect start to your day.

Cooking Time: 10 minutes

Servings: 2

Ingredients:

- 2 ripe avocados
- 4 slices of gluten-free bread
- 1 tablespoon fresh parsley, chopped
- 1 tablespoon fresh basil, chopped
- 1 tablespoon fresh chives, chopped
- Juice of 1/2 lemon
- Salt and pepper to taste

Instructions:

1. Toast the gluten-free bread slices to your desired level of crispiness.
2. While the bread is toasting, cut the avocados in half, remove the pits, and scoop the flesh into a bowl.
3. Mash the avocado with a fork until it reaches your preferred consistency.
4. Add the lemon juice, salt, and pepper to the mashed avocado, and mix well.
5. Spread the avocado mixture evenly over the toasted bread slices.
6. Sprinkle the chopped parsley, basil, and chives over the avocado toast.
7. Serve immediately and enjoy!

Tips:

- For extra flavor, drizzle a bit of olive oil over the top.
- Add a poached egg on top for additional protein.
- Experiment with different herbs to find your favorite combination.

Nutritional Info (per serving):

- Calories: 350
- Protein: 6g
- Carbohydrates: 30g
- Fat: 26g
- Fiber: 10g

* * *

Scrambled Eggs with Spinach

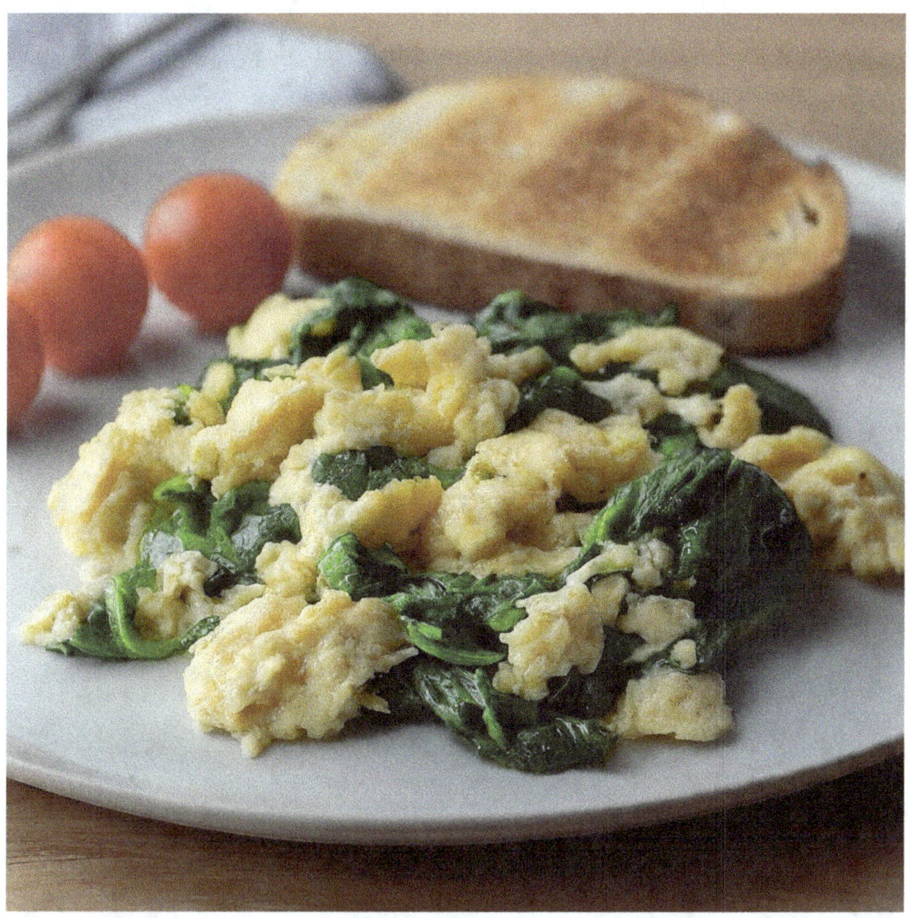

Scrambled Eggs with Spinach is a quick and nutritious breakfast that's high in protein and packed with vitamins. It's a great way to start your day with a balanced meal.

Cooking Time: 10 minutes

Servings: 2

Ingredients:

- 4 large eggs
- 1 cup fresh spinach, chopped
- 2 tablespoons olive oil or butter

- 1/4 cup unsweetened almond milk (or any low-histamine milk alternative)
- Salt and pepper to taste
- Fresh chives for garnish (optional)

Instructions:

1. In a medium bowl, whisk the eggs and almond milk together until well combined.
2. Heat the olive oil or butter in a non-stick skillet over medium heat.
3. Add the chopped spinach to the skillet and sauté for 1-2 minutes, until wilted.
4. Pour the egg mixture into the skillet with the spinach.
5. Cook, stirring gently, until the eggs are fully cooked and scrambled to your liking.
6. Season with salt and pepper to taste.
7. Garnish with fresh chives if desired.
8. Serve immediately and enjoy!

Tips:

- For a creamier texture, add a tablespoon of cream cheese to the eggs before cooking.
- Pair with a side of avocado or fresh fruit for a complete meal.
- Use baby spinach for a milder flavor.

Nutritional Info (per serving):

- Calories: 250
- Protein: 14g
- Carbohydrates: 4g
- Fat: 20g
- Fiber: 2g

Lunch Recipes

Quinoa and Cucumber Salad

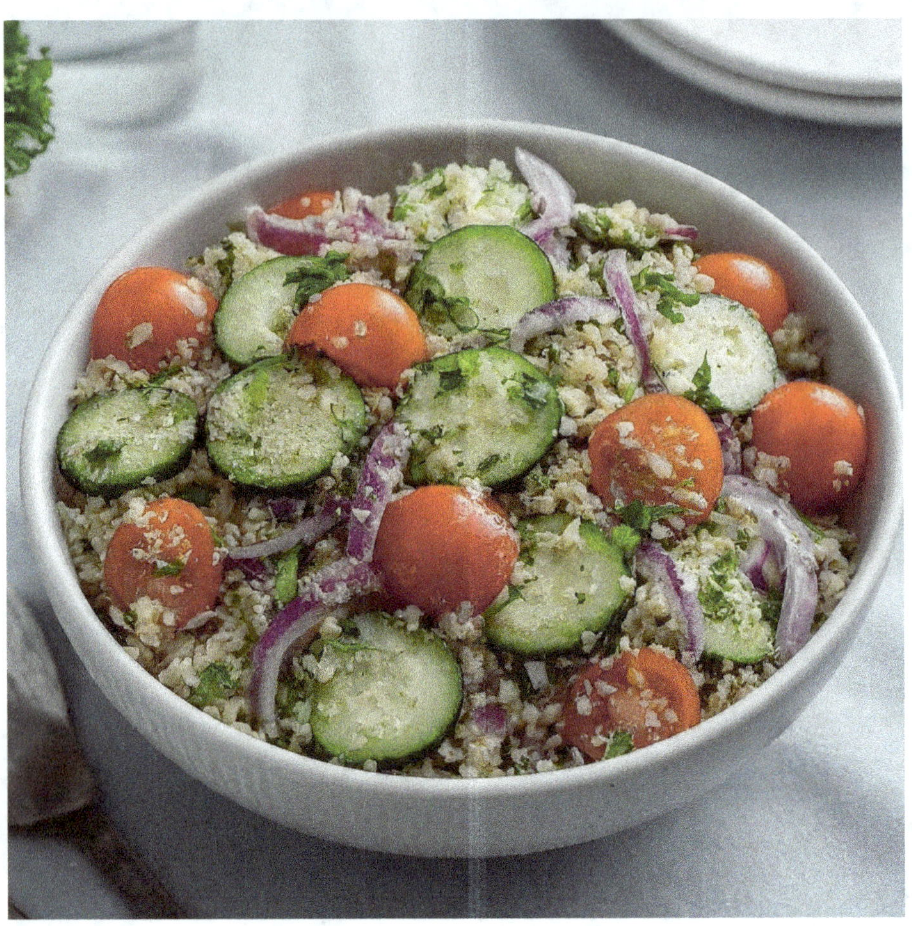

This Quinoa and Cucumber Salad is a light, refreshing, and nutritious meal perfect for a quick lunch. Packed with protein, fiber, and hydrating vegetables, it's both satisfying and healthy.

Cooking Time: 20 minutes

Servings: 4

Ingredients:

- 1 cup quinoa, rinsed
- 2 cups water
- 1 large cucumber, diced

- 1 cup cherry tomatoes, halved
- 1/4 cup fresh parsley, chopped
- 1/4 cup fresh mint, chopped
- Juice of 1 lemon
- 2 tablespoons olive oil
- Salt and pepper to taste

Instructions:

1. In a medium pot, bring the quinoa and water to a boil. Reduce heat to low, cover, and simmer for 15 minutes, or until the water is absorbed and the quinoa is tender.
2. Remove the quinoa from heat and let it cool for a few minutes.
3. In a large bowl, combine the cooked quinoa, cucumber, cherry tomatoes, parsley, and mint.
4. In a small bowl, whisk together the lemon juice, olive oil, salt, and pepper.
5. Pour the dressing over the quinoa mixture and toss to combine.
6. Serve immediately or refrigerate for an hour to allow flavors to meld.

Tips:

- Add diced avocado for extra creaminess.
- For added protein, include grilled chicken or chickpeas.
- This salad can be made ahead and stored in the fridge for up to 3 days.

Nutritional Info (per serving):

- Calories: 220
- Protein: 6g
- Carbohydrates: 32g
- Fat: 8g
- Fiber: 5g

* * *

Mixed Greens with Pear and Walnut

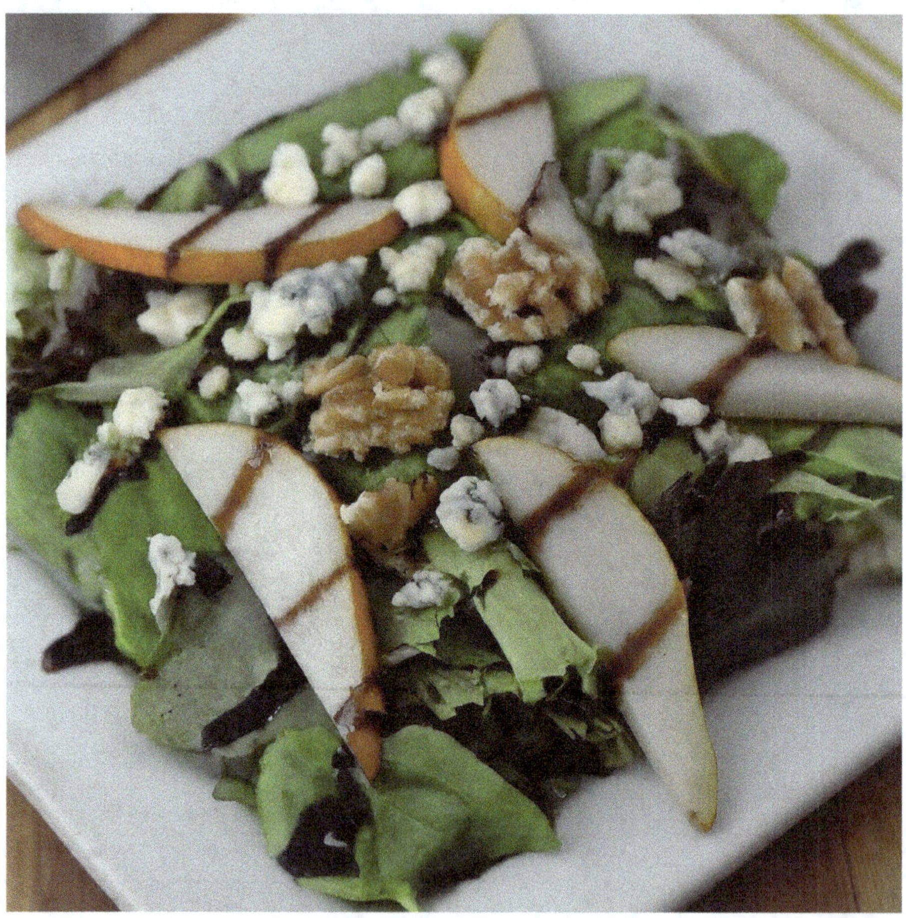

Mixed Greens with Pear and Walnut is a simple yet elegant salad that combines the sweetness of pears with the crunch of walnuts. It's a delightful and healthy lunch option.

Cooking Time: 10 minutes

Servings: 4

Ingredients:

- 4 cups mixed greens (spinach, arugula, and lettuce)
- 2 ripe pears, thinly sliced
- 1/2 cup walnuts, chopped
- 1/4 cup crumbled goat cheese (optional)
- 2 tablespoons olive oil
- 1 tablespoon apple cider vinegar
- 1 teaspoon honey (optional, if tolerated)
- Salt and pepper to taste

Instructions:

1. In a large bowl, combine the mixed greens, sliced pears, and walnuts.
2. If using, sprinkle the goat cheese over the salad.
3. In a small bowl, whisk together the olive oil, apple cider vinegar, honey, salt, and pepper.
4. Drizzle the dressing over the salad and toss gently to combine.
5. Serve immediately.

Tips:

- Toast the walnuts in a dry skillet for a few minutes to enhance their flavor.
- Substitute goat cheese with feta or leave it out for a dairy-free option.
- Add grilled chicken or tofu for extra protein.

Nutritional Info (per serving):

- Calories: 200
- Protein: 4g

- Carbohydrates: 18g
- Fat: 14g
- Fiber: 4g

40

* * *

Carrot Ginger Soup

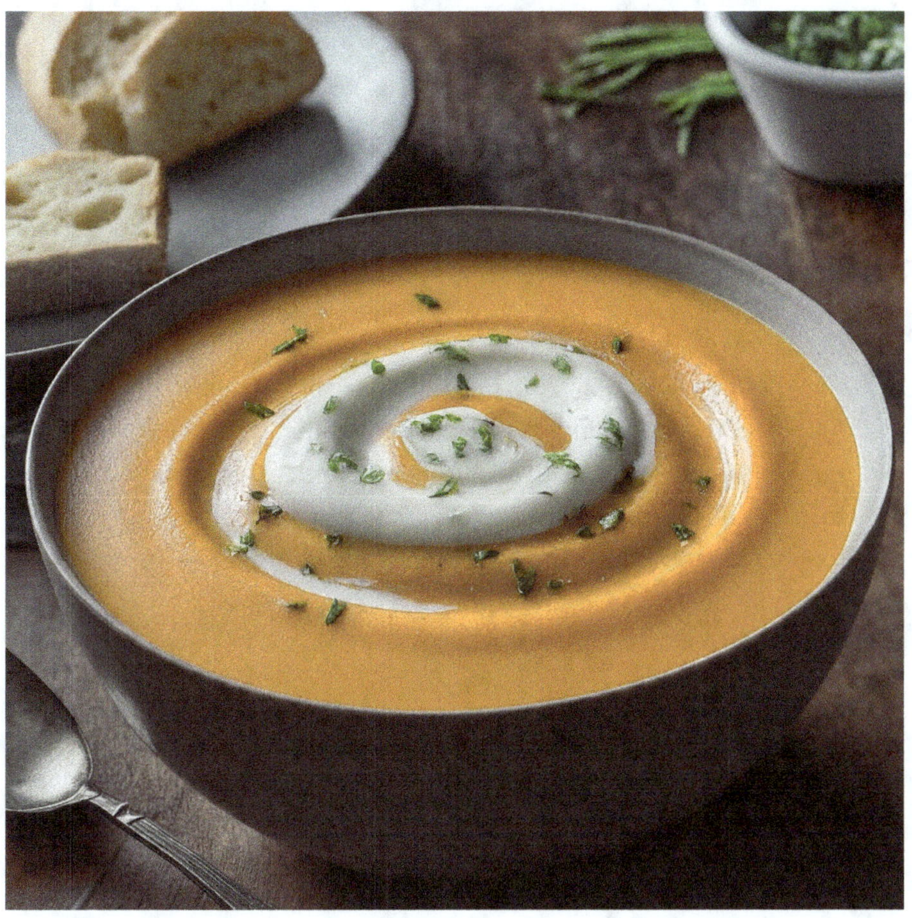

This Carrot Ginger Soup is a warming and comforting dish, perfect for a light lunch. The combination of carrots and ginger offers a vibrant flavor and a boost of nutrients.

Cooking Time: 30 minutes

Servings: 4

Ingredients:

- 1 tablespoon olive oil
- 1 onion, chopped
- 4 large carrots, peeled and chopped

- 1-inch piece of fresh ginger, peeled and grated
- 4 cups low-sodium vegetable broth
- Salt and pepper to taste
- Fresh parsley for garnish

Instructions:

1. In a large pot, heat the olive oil over medium heat.
2. Add the chopped onion and sauté until translucent, about 5 minutes.
3. Add the carrots and ginger, and cook for another 5 minutes.
4. Pour in the vegetable broth and bring to a boil. Reduce heat and simmer for 20 minutes, or until the carrots are tender.
5. Use an immersion blender to puree the soup until smooth, or transfer to a blender in batches.
6. Season with salt and pepper to taste.
7. Garnish with fresh parsley and serve hot.

Tips:

- For a creamier texture, add a splash of coconut milk before blending.
- Serve with a side of gluten-free bread for a complete meal.
- Adjust the amount of ginger to your taste preference.

Nutritional Info (per serving):

- Calories: 120
- Protein: 2g
- Carbohydrates: 20g
- Fat: 4g
- Fiber: 5g

* * *

Sweet Potato and Leek Soup

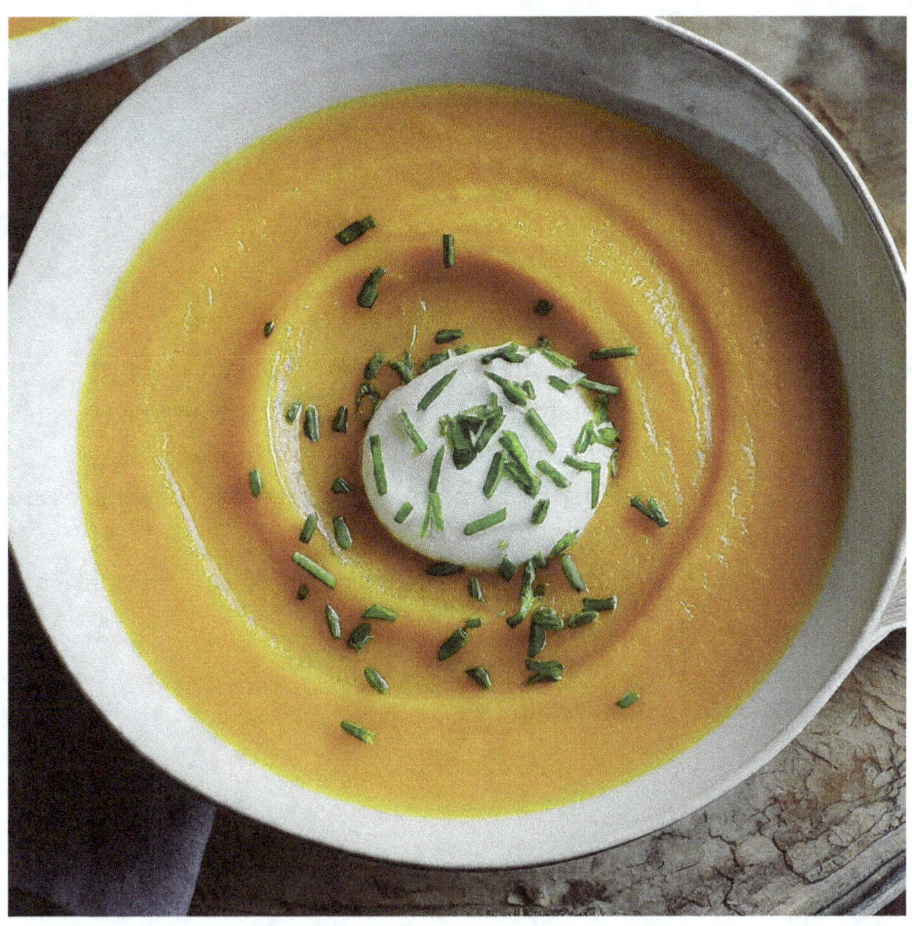

Sweet Potato and Leek Soup is a rich and velvety soup that's both nourishing and flavorful. It's an ideal dish for a cozy lunch or a light dinner.

Cooking Time: 35 minutes

Servings: 4

Ingredients:

- 2 tablespoons olive oil
- 2 leeks, white and light green parts only, sliced
- 2 large sweet potatoes, peeled and diced
- 4 cups low-sodium vegetable broth
- 1 teaspoon dried thyme
- Salt and pepper to taste
- Fresh chives for garnish

Instructions:

1. In a large pot, heat the olive oil over medium heat.
2. Add the sliced leeks and sauté until soft, about 5 minutes.
3. Add the diced sweet potatoes and cook for another 5 minutes.
4. Pour in the vegetable broth and add the thyme. Bring to a boil.
5. Reduce heat and simmer for 25 minutes, or until the sweet potatoes are tender.
6. Use an immersion blender to puree the soup until smooth, or transfer to a blender in batches.
7. Season with salt and pepper to taste.
8. Garnish with fresh chives and serve hot.

Tips:

- For extra creaminess, stir in a dollop of plain coconut yogurt before serving.
- Pair with a simple side salad for a well-rounded meal.
- Freeze leftovers in portioned containers for easy future meals.

Nutritional Info (per serving):

- Calories: 180
- Protein: 3g
- Carbohydrates: 30g

- Fat: 6g
- Fiber: 5g

45

* * *

Turkey and Avocado Wrap

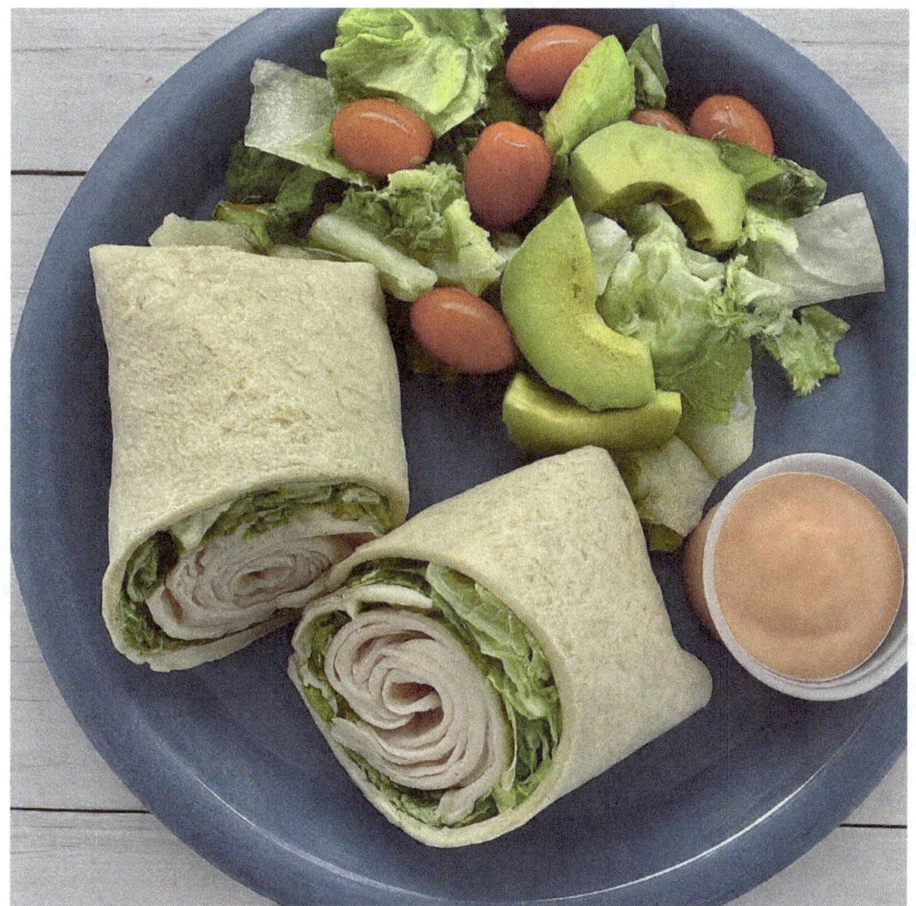

This Turkey and Avocado Wrap is a quick and easy lunch option that's both nutritious and satisfying. It combines lean turkey, creamy avocado, and fresh vegetables in a convenient wrap.

Cooking Time: 10 minutes

Servings: 2

Ingredients:

- 2 large gluten-free tortillas or wraps
- 1 ripe avocado, sliced
- 4 slices of cooked turkey breast (preferably freshly cooked)
- 1 cup fresh spinach leaves
- 1/2 cup shredded carrots
- 1/2 cup cucumber, sliced
- 2 tablespoons olive oil
- Juice of 1/2 lemon
- Salt and pepper to taste

Instructions:

1. In a small bowl, mix the olive oil, lemon juice, salt, and pepper to create a simple dressing.
2. Lay the gluten-free tortillas flat and evenly distribute the avocado slices on each.
3. Layer the turkey slices, spinach leaves, shredded carrots, and cucumber slices on top of the avocado.
4. Drizzle the dressing over the vegetables.
5. Roll up each tortilla tightly and slice in half.
6. Serve immediately or wrap in foil for an on-the-go lunch.

Tips:

- For added flavor, sprinkle with fresh herbs like cilantro or parsley.
- Use grilled chicken or roast beef as an alternative to turkey.

- Add a handful of sprouts for extra crunch and nutrition.

Nutritional Info (per serving):

- Calories: 350
- Protein: 18g
- Carbohydrates: 35g
- Fat: 18g
- Fiber: 8g

* * *

Grilled Chicken Sandwich with Homemade Mayo

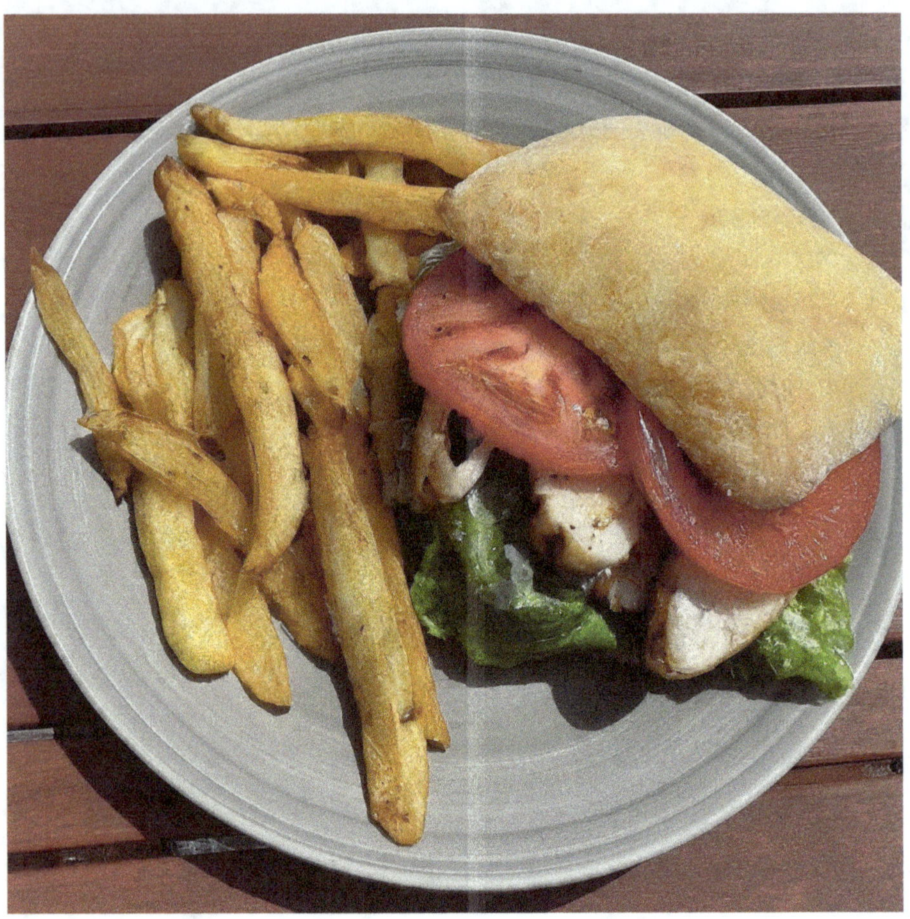

This Grilled Chicken Sandwich with Homemade Mayo is a hearty and delicious lunch option. The homemade mayo adds a rich, creamy touch without the preservatives found in store-bought versions.

Cooking Time: 20 minutes

Servings: 2

Ingredients:

- 2 boneless, skinless chicken breasts
- 2 gluten-free sandwich rolls or bread slices
- 1 ripe avocado, sliced

- 1 cup fresh lettuce leaves
- 1 tomato, sliced
- Salt and pepper to taste

For the Homemade Mayo:

- 1 large egg yolk
- 1 teaspoon Dijon mustard
- 1 tablespoon lemon juice
- 1/2 cup olive oil
- Salt and pepper to taste

Instructions:

1. **Grill the Chicken:**
2. Preheat your grill or grill pan to medium-high heat.
3. Season the chicken breasts with salt and pepper.
4. Grill the chicken for 6-7 minutes on each side, or until fully cooked and no longer pink in the center.
5. Remove from heat and let rest for a few minutes before slicing.
6. **Make the Homemade Mayo:**
7. In a medium bowl, whisk together the egg yolk, Dijon mustard, and lemon juice.
8. Slowly drizzle in the olive oil while continuously whisking until the mixture thickens and emulsifies.
9. Season with salt and pepper to taste.
10. **Assemble the Sandwich:**
11. Spread a generous layer of homemade mayo on the bottom half of each gluten-free roll or bread slice.
12. Layer the grilled chicken slices, avocado, lettuce, and tomato.
13. Top with the other half of the roll or bread slice.
14. Serve immediately.

Tips:

- For extra flavor, add a slice of low-histamine cheese like fresh mozzarella.
- Use the homemade mayo as a dip for veggies or a spread for other sandwiches.
- Grill extra chicken breasts and store them in the fridge for quick meals throughout the week.

Nutritional Info (per serving):

- Calories: 500
- Protein: 28g
- Carbohydrates: 35g
- Fat: 30g
- Fiber: 7g

Dinner Recipes

Baked Lemon Chicken with Roasted Vegetables

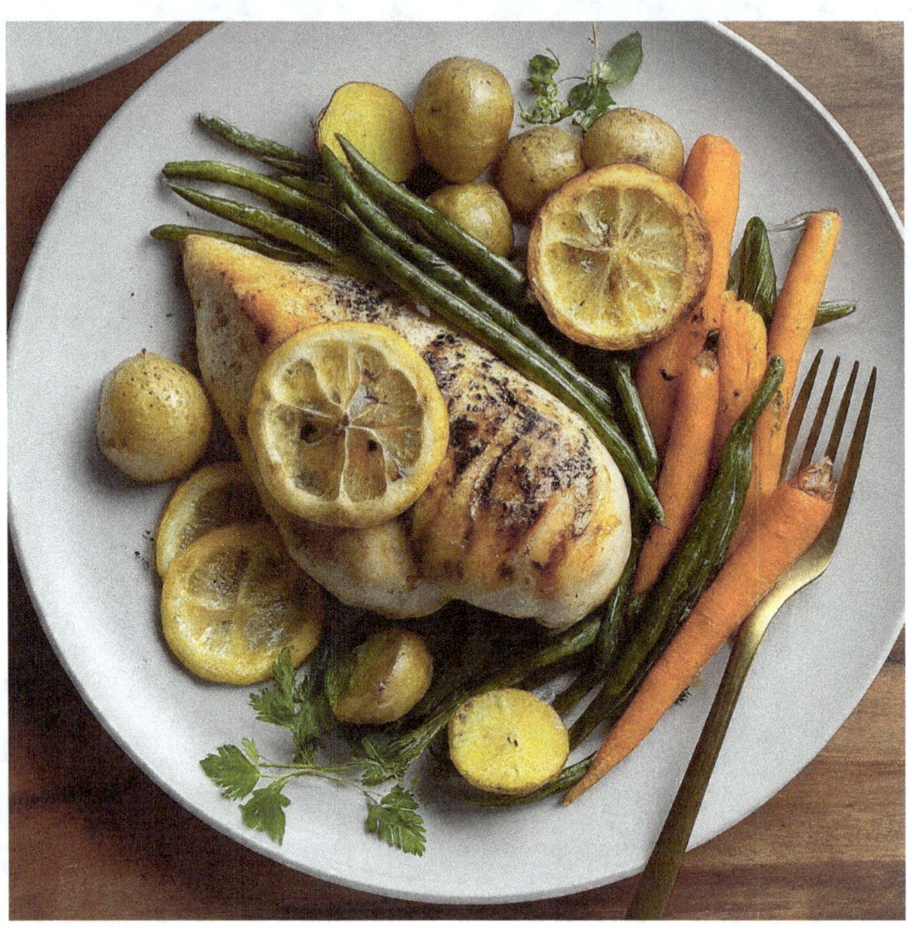

B aked Lemon Chicken with Roasted Vegetables is a healthy and flavorful dinner option. The lemon adds a refreshing zest to the tender chicken, while the roasted vegetables provide a colorful and nutritious side.

Cooking Time: 45 minutes

Servings: 4

Ingredients:

- 4 boneless, skinless chicken breasts
- 3 tablespoons olive oil

- Juice and zest of 1 lemon
- 3 garlic cloves, minced
- 1 teaspoon dried thyme
- 1 teaspoon dried rosemary
- Salt and pepper to taste
- 2 cups broccoli florets
- 2 cups carrots, chopped
- 2 cups bell peppers, chopped

Instructions:

1. Preheat your oven to 400°F (200°C).
2. In a small bowl, mix the olive oil, lemon juice, lemon zest, garlic, thyme, rosemary, salt, and pepper.
3. Place the chicken breasts in a baking dish and pour half of the lemon mixture over the chicken, coating evenly.
4. Arrange the broccoli, carrots, and bell peppers around the chicken in the baking dish.
5. Pour the remaining lemon mixture over the vegetables.
6. Bake for 30–35 minutes, or until the chicken is cooked through and the vegetables are tender.
7. Serve immediately, garnished with extra lemon zest if desired.

Tips:

- Marinate the chicken in the lemon mixture for a few hours for extra flavor.
- Substitute or add other vegetables like zucchini or asparagus.
- Serve with a side of quinoa or rice for a complete meal.

Nutritional Info (per serving):

- Calories: 350
- Protein: 30g

- Carbohydrates: 20g
- Fat: 15g
- Fiber: 6g

* * *

Beef Stir-Fry with Fresh Vegetables

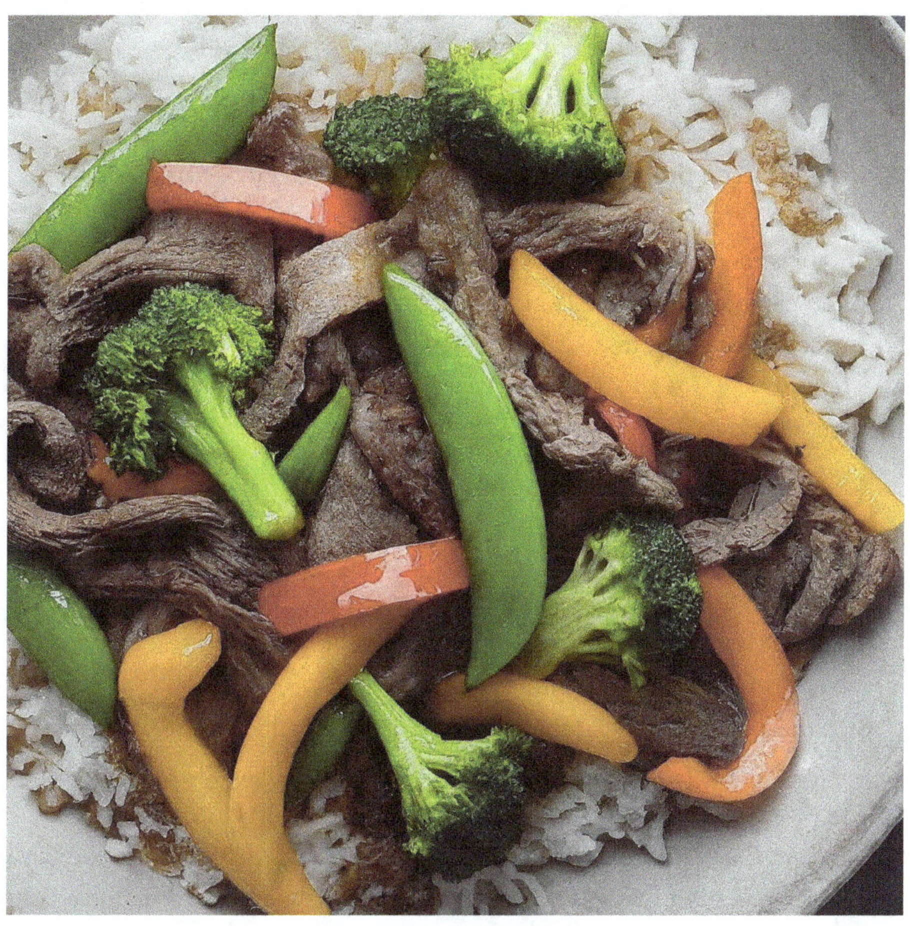

This Beef Stir-Fry with Fresh Vegetables is a quick and easy dinner that's both nutritious and delicious. The combination of tender beef and crisp vegetables makes for a satisfying meal.

Cooking Time: 30 minutes

Servings: 4

Ingredients:

- 1 lb (450g) beef sirloin, thinly sliced
- 3 tablespoons olive oil
- 3 garlic cloves, minced

- 1 tablespoon fresh ginger, grated
- 1 bell pepper, sliced
- 1 cup snap peas
- 1 cup broccoli florets
- 1 cup carrots, julienned
- 2 tablespoons coconut aminos (or low-histamine soy sauce alternative)
- 1 tablespoon cornstarch (optional, for thickening)
- Salt and pepper to taste

Instructions:

1. In a large skillet or wok, heat 2 tablespoons of olive oil over medium-high heat.
2. Add the garlic and ginger and sauté for 1 minute until fragrant.
3. Add the beef slices and cook until browned, about 5 minutes. Remove the beef from the skillet and set aside.
4. In the same skillet, add the remaining olive oil and the bell pepper, snap peas, broccoli, and carrots. Stir-fry for 5-7 minutes until the vegetables are tender-crisp.
5. Return the beef to the skillet and add the coconut aminos. Stir to combine.
6. If desired, dissolve the cornstarch in a small amount of water and add to the skillet to thicken the sauce.
7. Season with salt and pepper to taste and serve immediately.

Tips:

- Serve over a bed of rice or quinoa for a more filling meal.
- Adjust the vegetables to your liking or what you have on hand.
- Add a dash of hot sauce if you prefer a bit of spice.

Nutritional Info (per serving):

- Calories: 400

- Protein: 30g
- Carbohydrates: 15g
- Fat: 25g
- Fiber: 4g

* * *

Grilled Salmon with Quinoa

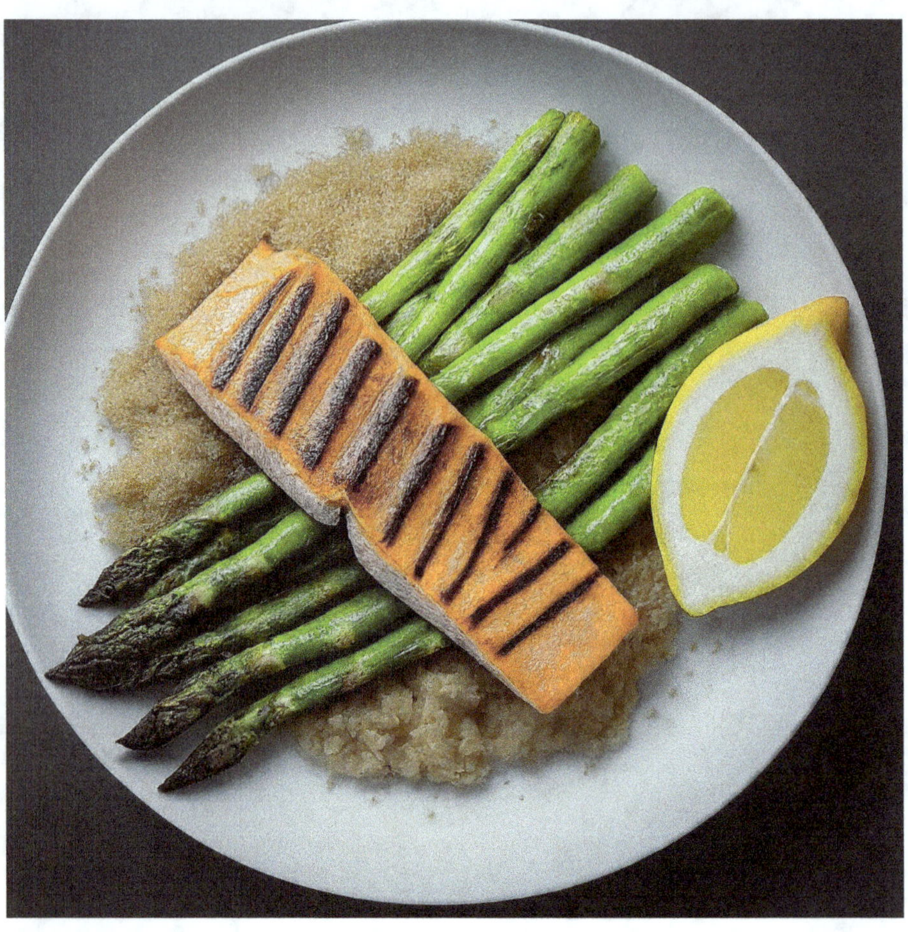

Grilled Salmon with Quinoa is a simple yet elegant dinner that's packed with protein and healthy fats. The quinoa provides a light and fluffy base, while the salmon is perfectly seasoned and grilled to perfection.

Cooking Time: 30 minutes

Servings: 4

Ingredients:

- 4 salmon fillets
- 2 tablespoons olive oil
- Juice of 1 lemon

- 2 garlic cloves, minced
- 1 teaspoon dried dill
- Salt and pepper to taste
- 1 cup quinoa, rinsed
- 2 cups water or low-sodium vegetable broth
- 1/4 cup fresh parsley, chopped

Instructions:

1. Preheat your grill to medium-high heat.
2. In a small bowl, mix the olive oil, lemon juice, garlic, dill, salt, and pepper.
3. Brush the salmon fillets with the mixture and let them marinate for 10 minutes.
4. In a medium pot, bring the quinoa and water or vegetable broth to a boil. Reduce heat to low, cover, and simmer for 15 minutes or until the quinoa is cooked and the liquid is absorbed.
5. Grill the salmon for 4-5 minutes per side, or until cooked to your desired doneness.
6. Fluff the cooked quinoa with a fork and stir in the fresh parsley.
7. Serve the grilled salmon on a bed of quinoa.

Tips:

- For extra flavor, marinate the salmon for up to 30 minutes.
- Serve with a side of steamed vegetables or a simple salad.
- Use leftover salmon in a salad or sandwich the next day.

Nutritional Info (per serving):

- Calories: 450
- Protein: 35g
- Carbohydrates: 30g
- Fat: 20g

· Fiber: 5g

* * *

Zucchini Noodles with Pesto

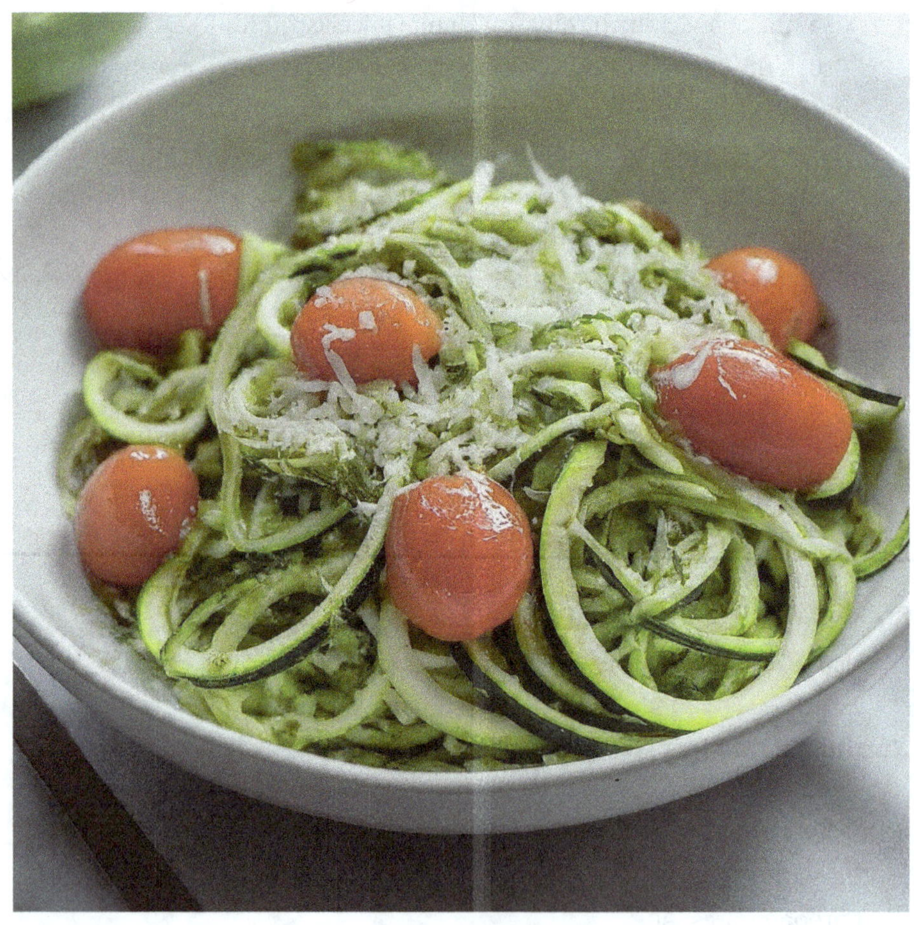

Zucchini Noodles with Pesto is a light and healthy dinner option that's perfect for those looking to reduce their carbohydrate intake. The fresh pesto sauce adds a burst of flavor to the zucchini noodles.

Cooking Time: 20 minutes

Servings: 4

Ingredients:

- 4 medium zucchinis, spiralized into noodles
- 2 cups fresh basil leaves
- 1/4 cup pine nuts
- 2 garlic cloves
- 1/2 cup olive oil
- 1/4 cup nutritional yeast (or Parmesan cheese if tolerated)
- Salt and pepper to taste
- Cherry tomatoes for garnish (optional)

Instructions:

1. In a food processor, combine the basil leaves, pine nuts, and garlic. Pulse until finely chopped.
2. With the processor running, slowly add the olive oil until the mixture is smooth and creamy.
3. Add the nutritional yeast (or Parmesan cheese) and pulse until combined. Season with salt and pepper to taste.
4. In a large skillet, heat a small amount of olive oil over medium heat.
5. Add the zucchini noodles and sauté for 3-4 minutes, until just tender.
6. Remove from heat and toss the zucchini noodles with the pesto sauce until evenly coated.
7. Garnish with cherry tomatoes if desired and serve immediately.

Tips:

- For added protein, top with grilled chicken or shrimp.

- Store any leftover pesto in an airtight container in the fridge for up to a week.
- Use a mix of zucchini and carrot noodles for extra color and nutrients.

Nutritional Info (per serving):

- Calories: 250
- Protein: 5g
- Carbohydrates: 10g
- Fat: 22g
- Fiber: 4g

* * *

Lentil and Vegetable Stew

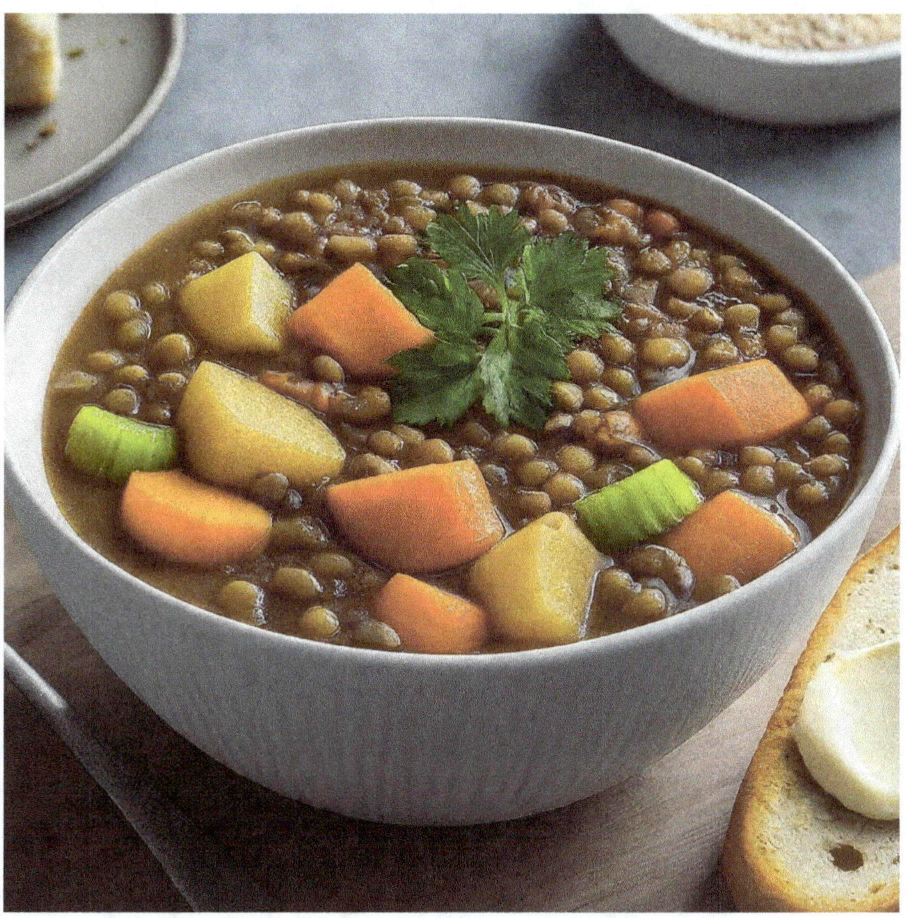

Lentil and Vegetable Stew is a hearty and comforting dish that's packed with protein, fiber, and a variety of nutrients. It's a perfect meal for a cozy dinner and can easily be made in large batches for meal prep.

Cooking Time: 45 minutes

Servings: 6

Ingredients:

- 2 tablespoons olive oil
- 1 onion, chopped
- 3 garlic cloves, minced

- 3 carrots, chopped
- 2 celery stalks, chopped
- 1 zucchini, chopped
- 1 bell pepper, chopped
- 1 cup dried lentils, rinsed
- 6 cups low-sodium vegetable broth
- 1 teaspoon dried thyme
- 1 teaspoon dried oregano
- 1 bay leaf
- Salt and pepper to taste
- Fresh parsley for garnish

Instructions:

- In a large pot, heat the olive oil over medium heat.
- Add the chopped onion and garlic, and sauté until the onion is translucent, about 5 minutes.
- Add the carrots, celery, zucchini, and bell pepper. Cook for another 5 minutes, stirring occasionally.
- Stir in the lentils, vegetable broth, thyme, oregano, and bay leaf.
- Bring to a boil, then reduce the heat and simmer for 30-35 minutes, or until the lentils and vegetables are tender.
- Remove the bay leaf and season with salt and pepper to taste.
- Garnish with fresh parsley before serving.

Tips:

- For added flavor, add a splash of lemon juice before serving.
- Use green or brown lentils, as they hold their shape better in stews.
- Serve with a side of crusty gluten-free bread for a complete meal.

Nutritional Info (per serving):

- Calories: 250
- Protein: 12g
- Carbohydrates: 40g
- Fat: 6g
- Fiber: 15g

* * *

Chicken and Rice Casserole

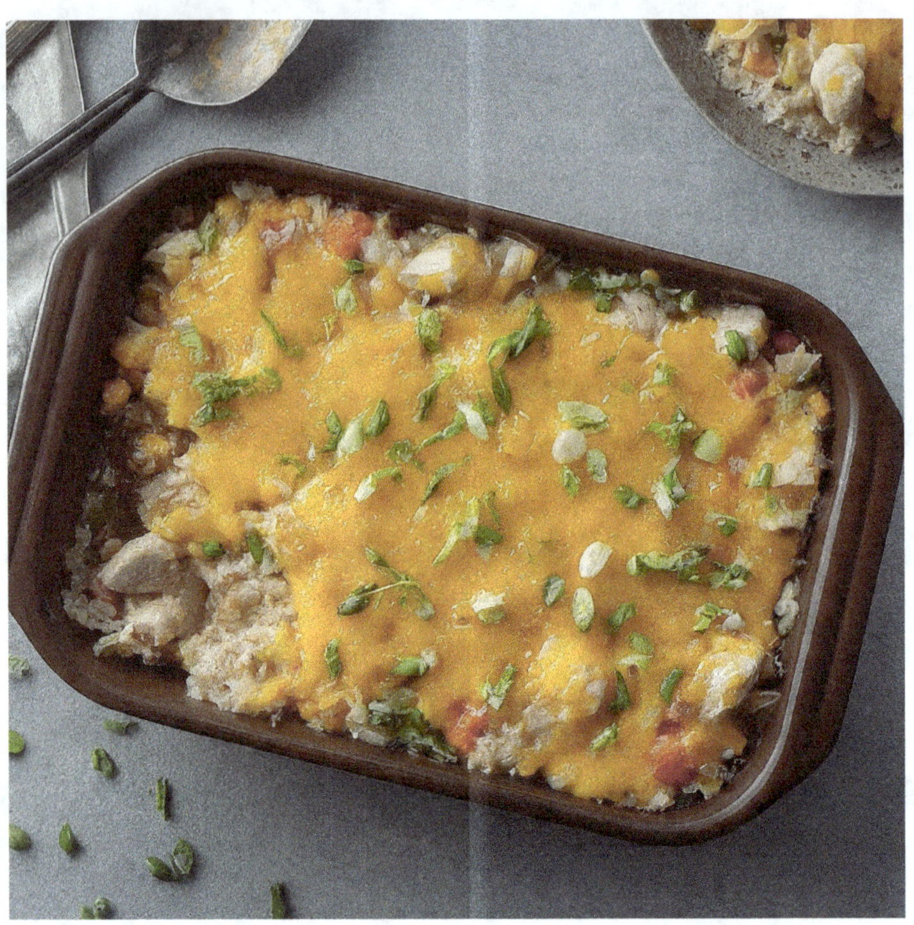

Chicken and Rice Casserole is a classic comfort food dish that's easy to prepare and perfect for a family dinner. This recipe combines tender chicken, fluffy rice, and a mix of vegetables for a well-rounded meal.

Cooking Time: 1 hour

Servings: 6

Ingredients:

- 2 tablespoons olive oil
- 1 onion, chopped
- 2 garlic cloves, minced

- 2 cups uncooked brown rice
- 4 cups low-sodium chicken broth
- 4 boneless, skinless chicken breasts
- 1 cup carrots, chopped
- 1 cup peas (fresh or frozen)
- 1 teaspoon dried thyme
- 1 teaspoon dried rosemary
- Salt and pepper to taste
- Fresh parsley for garnish

Instructions:

- Preheat your oven to 375°F (190°C).
- In a large oven-safe skillet or casserole dish, heat the olive oil over medium heat.
- Add the chopped onion and garlic, and sauté until the onion is translucent, about 5 minutes.
- Stir in the brown rice and cook for 1-2 minutes until slightly toasted.
- Add the chicken broth, carrots, peas, thyme, rosemary, salt, and pepper.
- Nestle the chicken breasts into the rice mixture.
- Bring the mixture to a boil, then cover the skillet or casserole dish with a lid or aluminum foil.
- Transfer to the preheated oven and bake for 45 minutes, or until the rice is cooked and the chicken is tender.
- Remove from the oven and let it sit for 5 minutes before serving.
- Garnish with fresh parsley before serving.

Tips:

- For extra flavor, marinate the chicken breasts in lemon juice and herbs before cooking.
- Substitute brown rice with white rice if preferred, but adjust cooking time accordingly.

- Add other vegetables like bell peppers or zucchini for variety.

Nutritional Info (per serving):

- Calories: 400
- Protein: 30g
- Carbohydrates: 50g
- Fat: 10g
- Fiber: 6g

Snacks and Appetizers

Fresh Fruit Salad

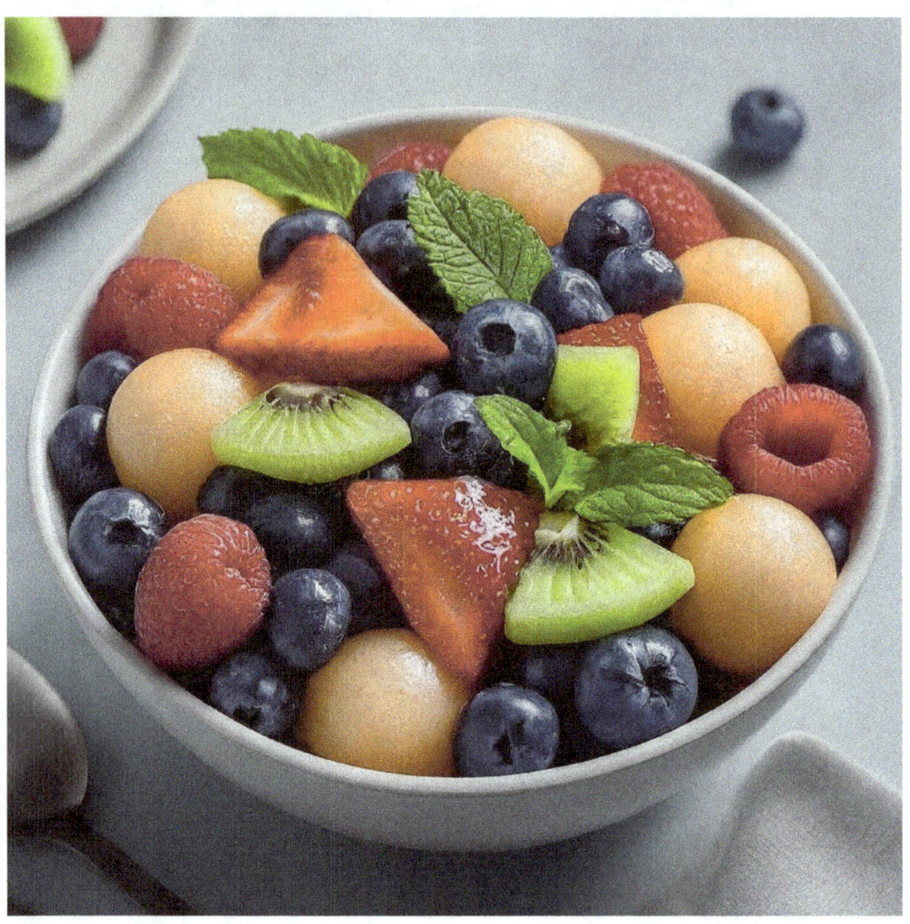

Fresh Fruit Salad is a simple and refreshing snack that's perfect for any time of the day. Packed with a variety of fruits, it's both delicious and nutritious, providing a healthy dose of vitamins and fiber.

Cooking Time: 15 minutes

Servings: 4

Ingredients:

- 1 cup strawberries, hulled and sliced
- 1 cup blueberries
- 1 cup pineapple, diced

- 1 apple, cored and diced
- 1 banana, sliced
- Juice of 1/2 lemon
- 1 tablespoon honey (optional, if tolerated)

Instructions:

1. In a large bowl, combine the strawberries, blueberries, pineapple, apple, and banana.
2. Drizzle the lemon juice over the fruit and toss gently to combine.
3. If using, drizzle honey over the salad and mix well.
4. Serve immediately or refrigerate for up to 2 hours before serving.

Tips:

- Use any combination of your favorite low-histamine fruits.
- Add a handful of fresh mint leaves for extra flavor.
- Serve with a dollop of coconut yogurt for added creaminess.

Nutritional Info (per serving):

- Calories: 100
- Protein: 1g
- Carbohydrates: 25g
- Fat: 0g
- Fiber: 5g

* * *

Rice Cakes with Almond Butter

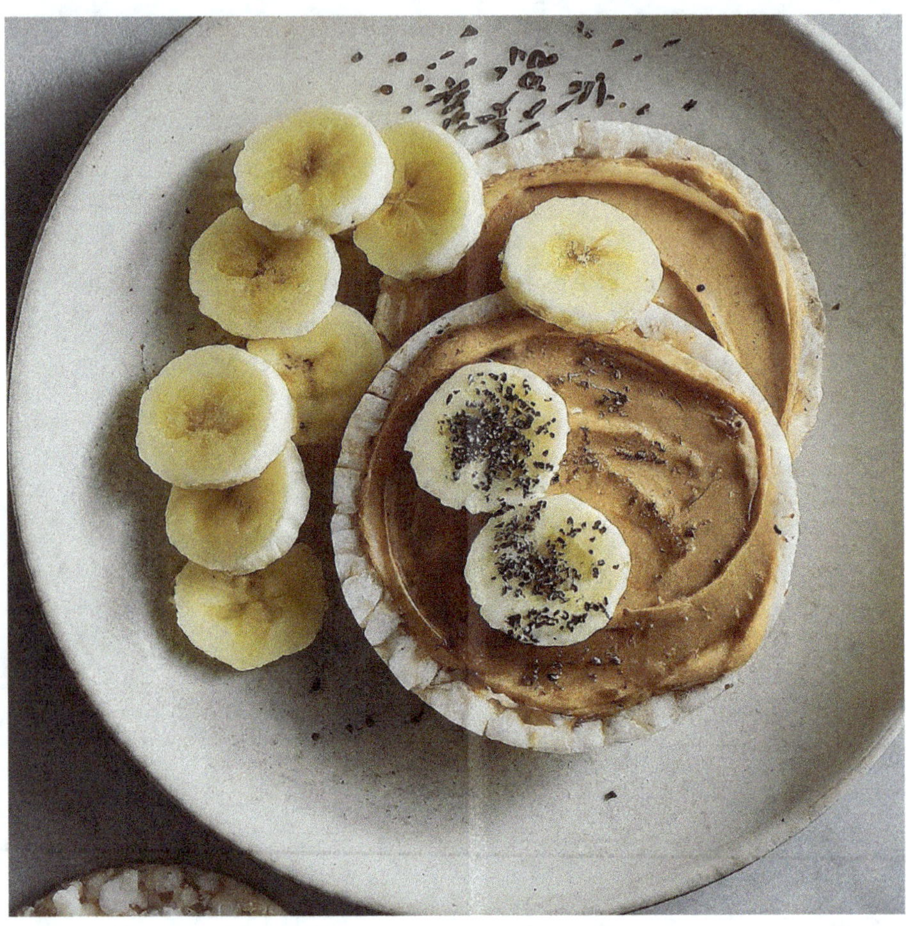

Rice Cakes with Almond Butter are a quick and easy snack that's perfect for a boost of energy. The combination of crunchy rice cakes and creamy almond butter is satisfying and nutritious.

Cooking Time: 5 minutes

Servings: 2

Ingredients:

- 4 rice cakes (ensure they are gluten-free and low in histamine)
- 4 tablespoons almond butter (ensure it is plain and low in histamine)
- 1 banana, sliced (optional)
- Drizzle of honey (optional, if tolerated)

Instructions:

1. Spread 1 tablespoon of almond butter on each rice cake.
2. Top with banana slices if using.
3. Drizzle with honey if desired.
4. Serve immediately.

Tips:

- Use sunflower seed butter or coconut butter as an alternative if almond butter is not tolerated.
- Sprinkle with chia seeds or flaxseeds for extra nutrition.
- Pair with a glass of almond milk for a more filling snack.

Nutritional Info (per serving):

- Calories: 250
- Protein: 6g
- Carbohydrates: 30g
- Fat: 12g
- Fiber: 4g

* * *

Guacamole with Veggie Sticks

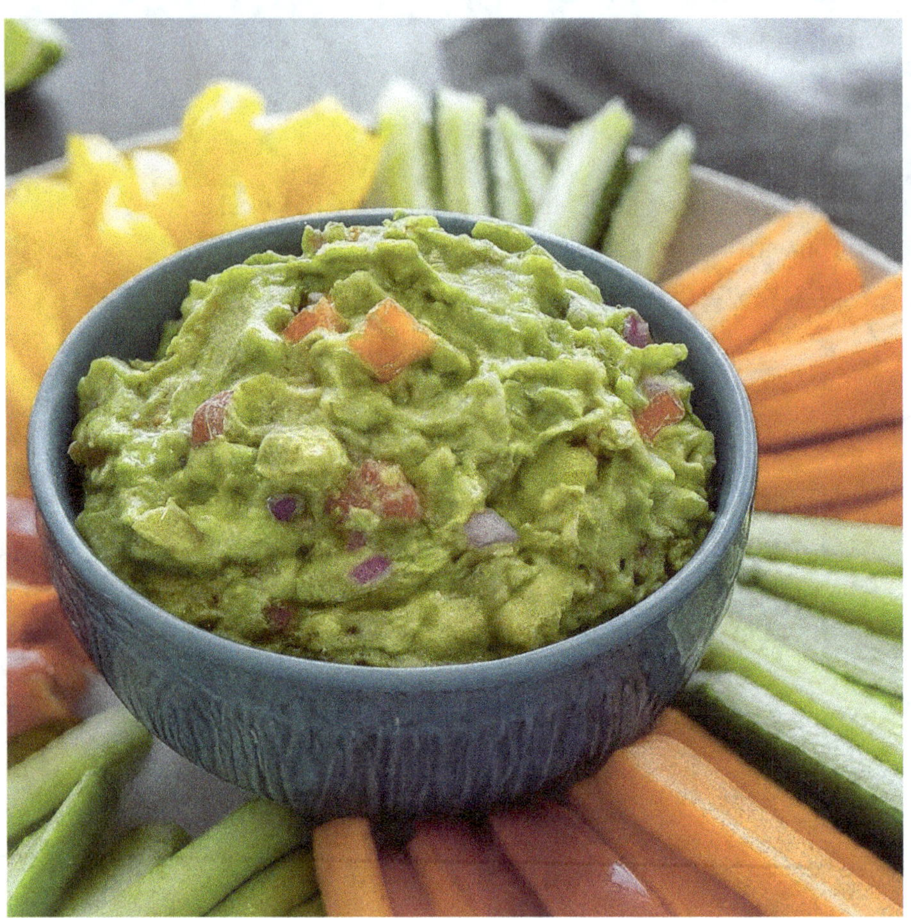

Guacamole with Veggie Sticks is a delicious and healthy snack that's perfect for dipping. The creamy guacamole pairs perfectly with crunchy vegetables, making it a great choice for a light snack or appetizer.

Cooking Time: 15 minutes

Servings: 4

Ingredients:

- 2 ripe avocados
- 1 small tomato, finely chopped
- 1/4 cup red onion, finely chopped
- Juice of 1 lime
- 2 tablespoons fresh cilantro, chopped
- Salt and pepper to taste
- Veggie sticks (carrots, celery, bell peppers, cucumber) for serving

Instructions:

1. In a medium bowl, mash the avocados until smooth.
2. Add the chopped tomato, red onion, lime juice, cilantro, salt, and pepper.
3. Mix well until all ingredients are combined.
4. Serve the guacamole with an assortment of veggie sticks.

Tips:

- For a spicier version, add a finely chopped jalapeño.
- Keep the avocado pits in the guacamole to prevent browning if storing.
- Use the guacamole as a spread for sandwiches or wraps.

Nutritional Info (per serving):

- Calories: 180
- Protein: 2g
- Carbohydrates: 12g
- Fat: 15g
- Fiber: 8g

* * *

Hummus with Gluten-Free Crackers

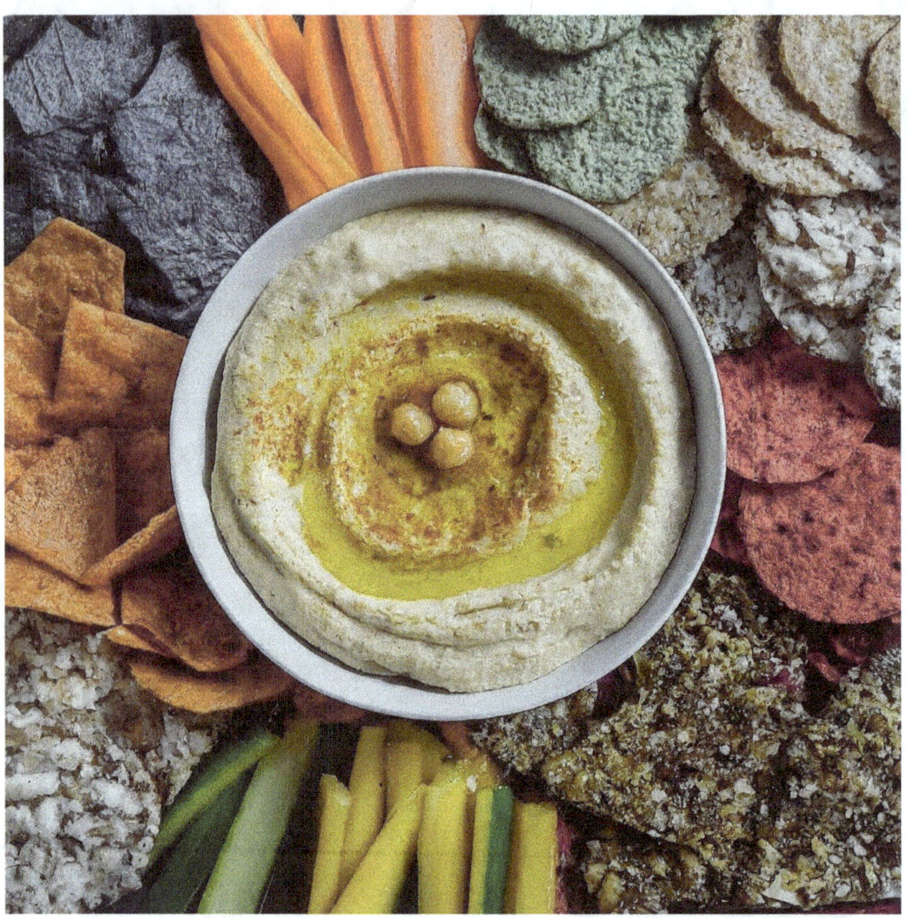

Hummus with Gluten-Free Crackers is a satisfying and protein-rich snack. The creamy hummus pairs perfectly with crunchy crackers, making it a great option for a quick and healthy bite.

Cooking Time: 10 minutes

Servings: 4

Ingredients:

- 1 can (15 oz) chickpeas, drained and rinsed
- 1/4 cup tahini
- 2 tablespoons olive oil
- Juice of 1 lemon
- 1 garlic clove, minced
- 1/2 teaspoon cumin
- Salt and pepper to taste
- 1/4 cup water (as needed for desired consistency)
- Gluten-free crackers for serving

Instructions:

1. In a food processor, combine the chickpeas, tahini, olive oil, lemon juice, garlic, cumin, salt, and pepper.
2. Blend until smooth, adding water as needed to reach the desired consistency.
3. Transfer the hummus to a bowl and serve with gluten-free crackers.

Tips:

- For a flavor twist, add roasted red peppers or sun-dried tomatoes to the hummus.
- Store leftover hummus in an airtight container in the fridge for up to a week.
- Use the hummus as a spread for sandwiches or as a dip for fresh vegetables.

Nutritional Info (per serving):

- Calories: 220
- Protein: 5g
- Carbohydrates: 20g
- Fat: 12g
- Fiber: 6g

Desserts

Coconut Macaroons

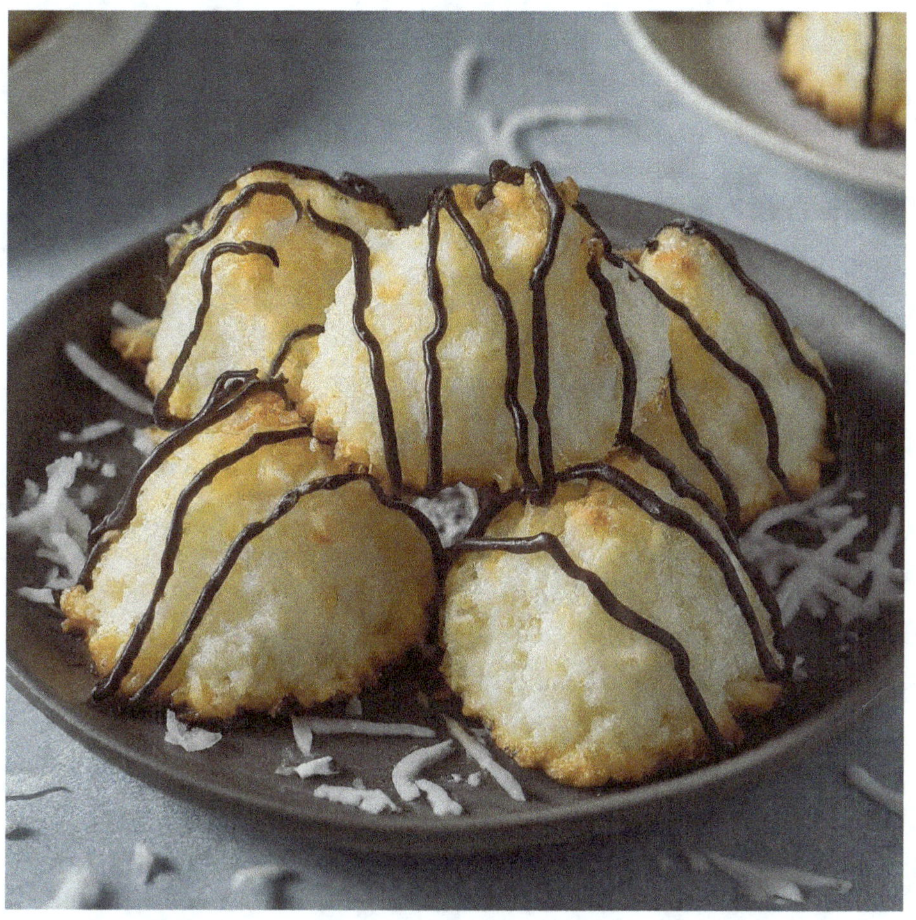

Coconut Macaroons are a delightful treat that's both chewy and crispy. Made with simple ingredients, these macaroons are naturally sweetened and perfect for satisfying your sweet tooth.

Cooking Time: 25 minutes

Servings: 12 macaroons

Ingredients:

- 2 1/2 cups unsweetened shredded coconut
- 1/2 cup almond flour
- 1/2 cup maple syrup or honey (if tolerated)

- 1/4 cup coconut oil, melted
- 1 teaspoon vanilla extract
- Pinch of salt

Instructions:

1. Preheat your oven to 325°F (160°C) and line a baking sheet with parchment paper.
2. In a large bowl, mix together the shredded coconut, almond flour, maple syrup, melted coconut oil, vanilla extract, and salt until well combined.
3. Using a tablespoon or a small cookie scoop, drop mounds of the mixture onto the prepared baking sheet.
4. Bake for 15–20 minutes, or until the edges are golden brown.
5. Let the macaroons cool on the baking sheet for 5 minutes before transferring to a wire rack to cool completely.
6. Store in an airtight container at room temperature.

Tips:

- For an extra touch, dip the bottoms of the macaroons in melted dark chocolate (if tolerated).
- Ensure the coconut oil is fully melted to help the ingredients bind together.
- These macaroons can be stored in the refrigerator for up to a week.

Nutritional Info (per serving):

- Calories: 150
- Protein: 2g
- Carbohydrates: 15g
- Fat: 10g
- Fiber: 3g

* * *

Fresh Berry Parfait

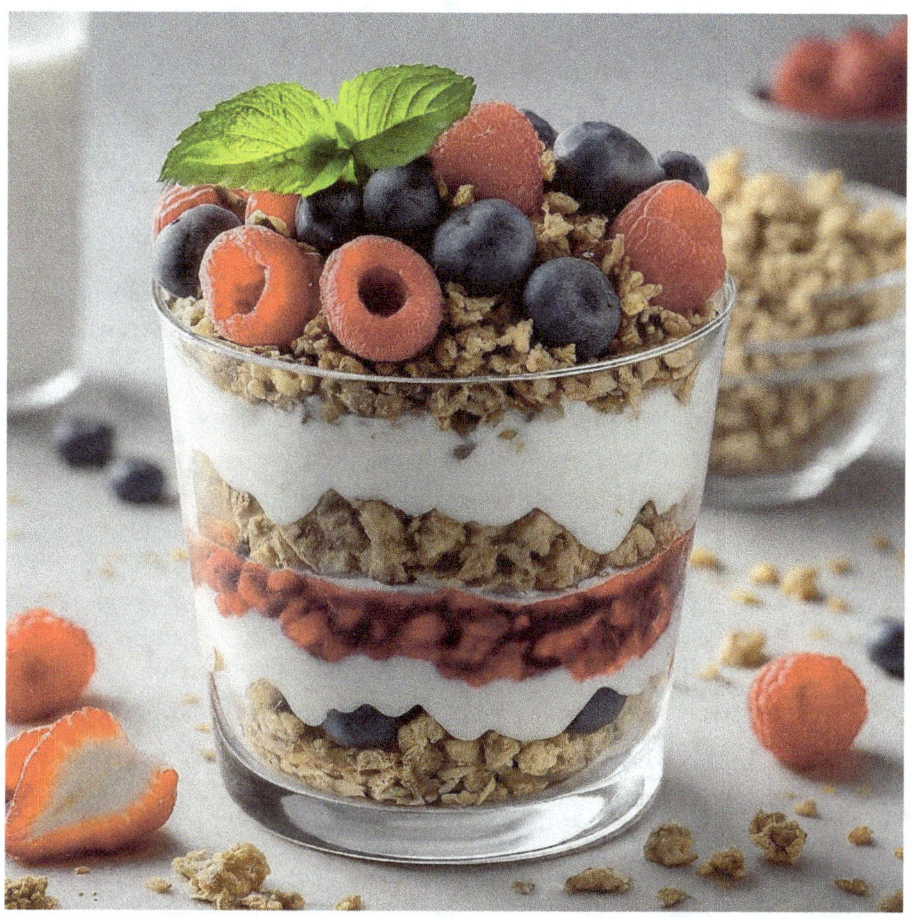

Fresh Berry Parfait is a light and refreshing dessert that's easy to assemble. It combines layers of fresh berries with creamy coconut yogurt for a naturally sweet and satisfying treat.

Cooking Time: 10 minutes

Servings: 4

Ingredients:

- 2 cups fresh strawberries, sliced
- 1 cup fresh blueberries
- 1 cup fresh raspberries
- 2 cups coconut yogurt (unsweetened)
- 1/4 cup granola (optional, ensure it's low-histamine and gluten-free)
- Fresh mint leaves for garnish

Instructions:

1. In four serving glasses or bowls, layer the coconut yogurt, strawberries, blueberries, and raspberries.
2. Repeat the layers until all ingredients are used up.
3. Top each parfait with a sprinkle of granola if using.
4. Garnish with fresh mint leaves and serve immediately.

Tips:

- Use any combination of your favorite low-histamine fruits.
- For added sweetness, drizzle a bit of honey or maple syrup over the parfait.
- These parfaits can also be made in advance and stored in the refrigerator for up to 2 hours before serving.

Nutritional Info (per serving):

- Calories: 180
- Protein: 3g
- Carbohydrates: 30g
- Fat: 7g

- Fiber: 7g

***

Banana Bread

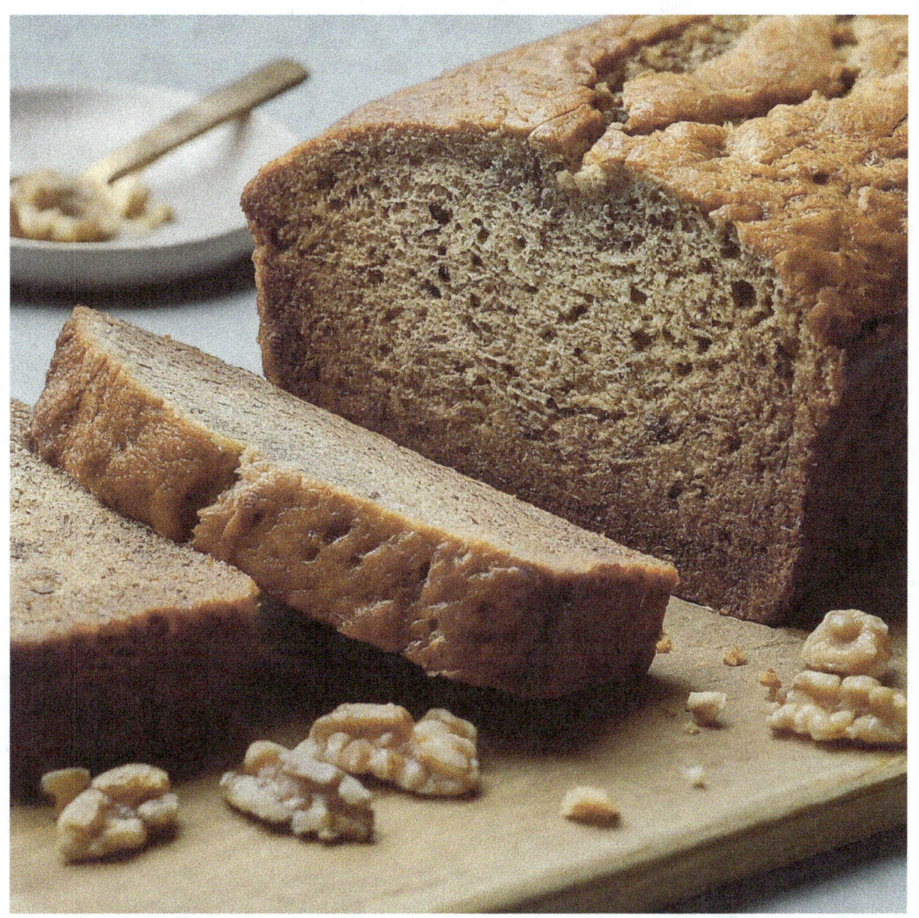

Banana Bread is a classic and comforting dessert that's easy to make and perfect for using up ripe bananas. This version is moist, flavorful, and made with simple ingredients.

Cooking Time: 1 hour

Servings: 8

Ingredients:

- 3 ripe bananas, mashed
- 1/3 cup coconut oil, melted
- 1/2 cup maple syrup or honey (if tolerated)
- 2 large eggs
- 1 teaspoon vanilla extract
- 1 teaspoon baking soda
- Pinch of salt
- 1 1/2 cups gluten-free flour blend

Instructions:

1. Preheat your oven to 350°F (175°C) and grease a loaf pan or line it with parchment paper.
2. In a large bowl, mix the mashed bananas, melted coconut oil, and maple syrup until well combined.
3. Add the eggs and vanilla extract, and mix until smooth.
4. Stir in the baking soda and salt.
5. Gradually add the gluten-free flour, mixing until just combined.
6. Pour the batter into the prepared loaf pan.
7. Bake for 50-60 minutes, or until a toothpick inserted into the center comes out clean.
8. Let the banana bread cool in the pan for 10 minutes before transferring to a wire rack to cool completely.
9. Slice and serve.

Tips:

- Add a handful of chopped nuts or chocolate chips to the batter for extra texture and flavor.
- Store the banana bread in an airtight container at room temperature for up to 3 days.
- This bread also freezes well; wrap slices individually for a quick treat.

Nutritional Info (per serving):

- Calories: 250
- Protein: 4g
- Carbohydrates: 40g
- Fat: 10g
- Fiber: 3g

* * *

Apple Cinnamon Muffins

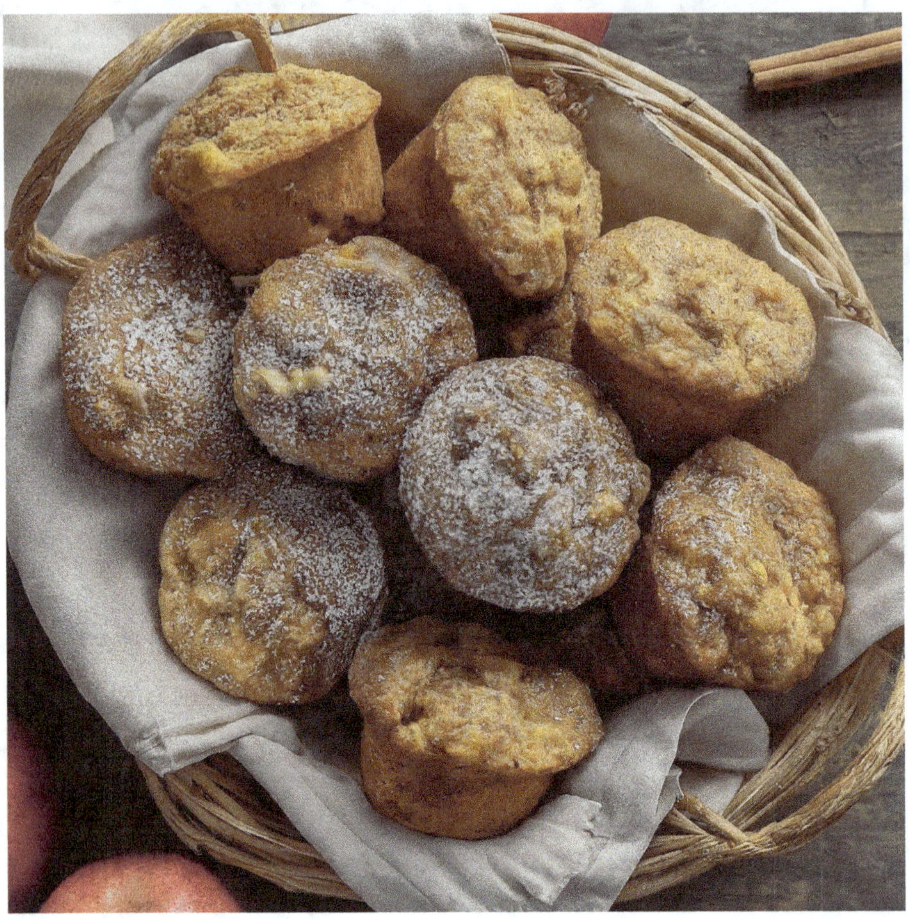

Apple Cinnamon Muffins are a warm and cozy treat that's perfect for breakfast or dessert. These muffins are moist, flavorful, and filled with chunks of fresh apple and warm spices.

Cooking Time: 30 minutes

Servings: 12 muffins

Ingredients:

- 2 cups gluten-free flour blend
- 1 teaspoon baking powder
- 1/2 teaspoon baking soda

- 1/2 teaspoon salt
- 1 teaspoon ground cinnamon
- 1/2 cup coconut oil, melted
- 1/2 cup maple syrup or honey (if tolerated)
- 2 large eggs
- 1 teaspoon vanilla extract
- 1 cup unsweetened applesauce
- 1 large apple, peeled and diced

Instructions:

1. Preheat your oven to 350°F (175°C) and line a muffin tin with paper liners.
2. In a large bowl, whisk together the gluten-free flour, baking powder, baking soda, salt, and cinnamon.
3. In a separate bowl, mix the melted coconut oil, maple syrup, eggs, vanilla extract, and applesauce until well combined.
4. Add the wet ingredients to the dry ingredients and mix until just combined.
5. Fold in the diced apple.
6. Divide the batter evenly among the muffin cups.
7. Bake for 20-25 minutes, or until a toothpick inserted into the center of a muffin comes out clean.
8. Let the muffins cool in the tin for 5 minutes before transferring to a wire rack to cool completely.

Tips:

- Sprinkle the tops of the muffins with a little extra cinnamon before baking for added flavor.
- These muffins can be stored in an airtight container at room temperature for up to 3 days.
- Freeze any leftover muffins for a quick and easy snack.

Nutritional Info (per serving):

- Calories: 200
- Protein: 3g
- Carbohydrates: 30g
- Fat: 8g
- Fiber: 3g

Drinks and Beverages

Herbal Iced Tea

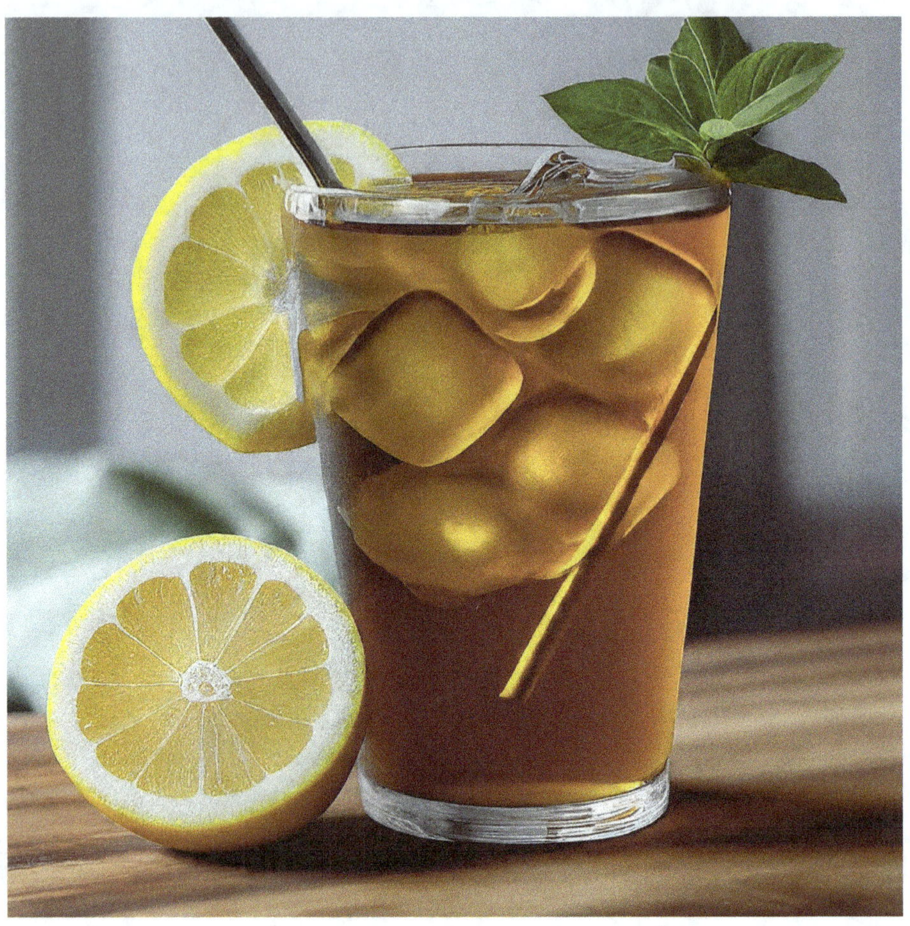

H erbal Iced Tea is a refreshing and caffeine-free drink perfect for hot days. Using a blend of your favorite herbal teas, this drink is hydrating and can be easily customized to your taste.

Cooking Time: 15 minutes (plus chilling time)

Servings: 4

Ingredients:

- 4 cups water
- 4 herbal tea bags (chamomile, peppermint, rooibos, or a blend)
- 1 tablespoon honey or maple syrup (optional, if tolerated)

- 1 lemon, sliced
- Fresh mint leaves for garnish
- Ice cubes

Instructions:

1. Bring the water to a boil in a large pot.
2. Remove from heat and add the herbal tea bags. Let steep for 5-7 minutes.
3. Remove the tea bags and stir in the honey or maple syrup if using.
4. Let the tea cool to room temperature, then transfer to a pitcher and refrigerate until cold.
5. Serve the iced tea over ice cubes, garnished with lemon slices and fresh mint leaves.

Tips:

- Experiment with different herbal tea blends to find your favorite flavor combination.
- Add a splash of fresh fruit juice (like apple or berry) for extra flavor.
- Make a big batch and store it in the refrigerator for up to a week.

Nutritional Info (per serving):

- Calories: 20 (without sweetener)
- Protein: 0g
- Carbohydrates: 5g
- Fat: 0g
- Fiber: 0g

* * *

Coconut Water with Lime

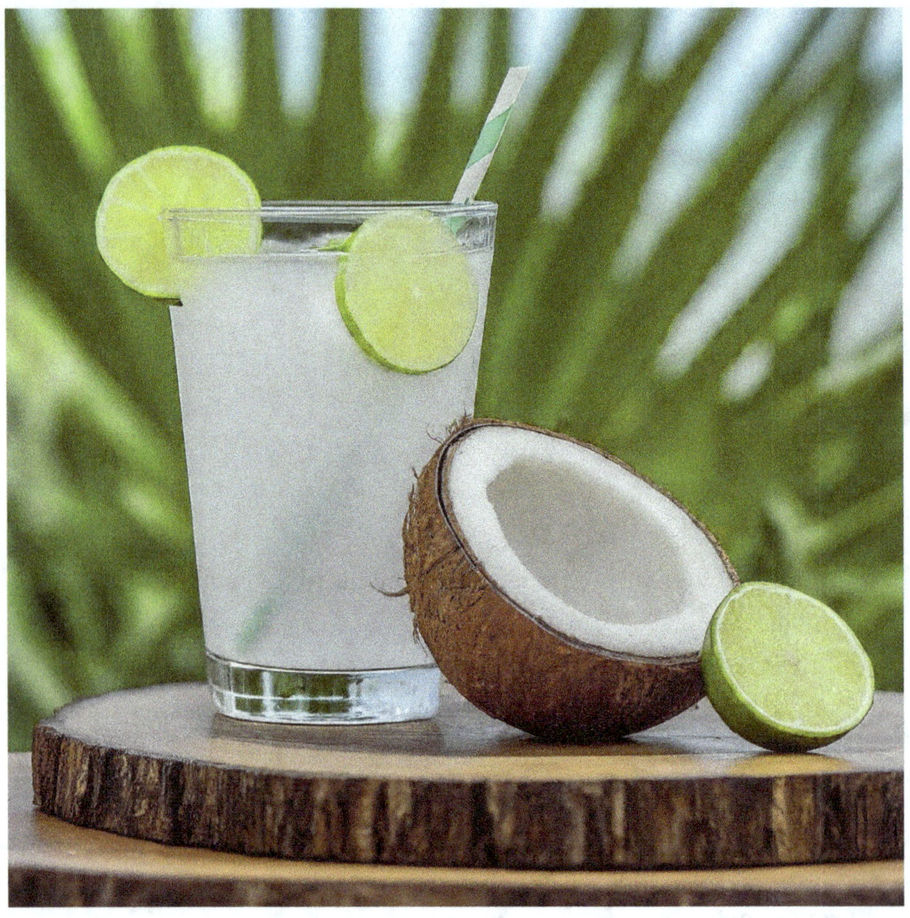

Coconut Water with Lime is a simple and hydrating drink that's perfect for rehydrating and refreshing your body. The natural electrolytes in coconut water make it an excellent choice for staying hydrated.

Cooking Time: 5 minutes

Servings: 2

Ingredients:

- 2 cups coconut water (unsweetened)
- Juice of 1 lime
- Lime slices for garnish
- Ice cubes

Instructions:

1. In a pitcher, combine the coconut water and lime juice.
2. Stir well to mix.
3. Serve over ice cubes and garnish with lime slices.

Tips:

- For added flavor, muddle some fresh mint leaves in the bottom of the glass before adding the coconut water and lime.
- Adjust the lime juice to your taste preference.
- Use chilled coconut water for an extra refreshing drink.

Nutritional Info (per serving):

- Calories: 45
- Protein: 0g
- Carbohydrates: 11g
- Fat: 0g
- Fiber: 0g

* * *

Turmeric Latte

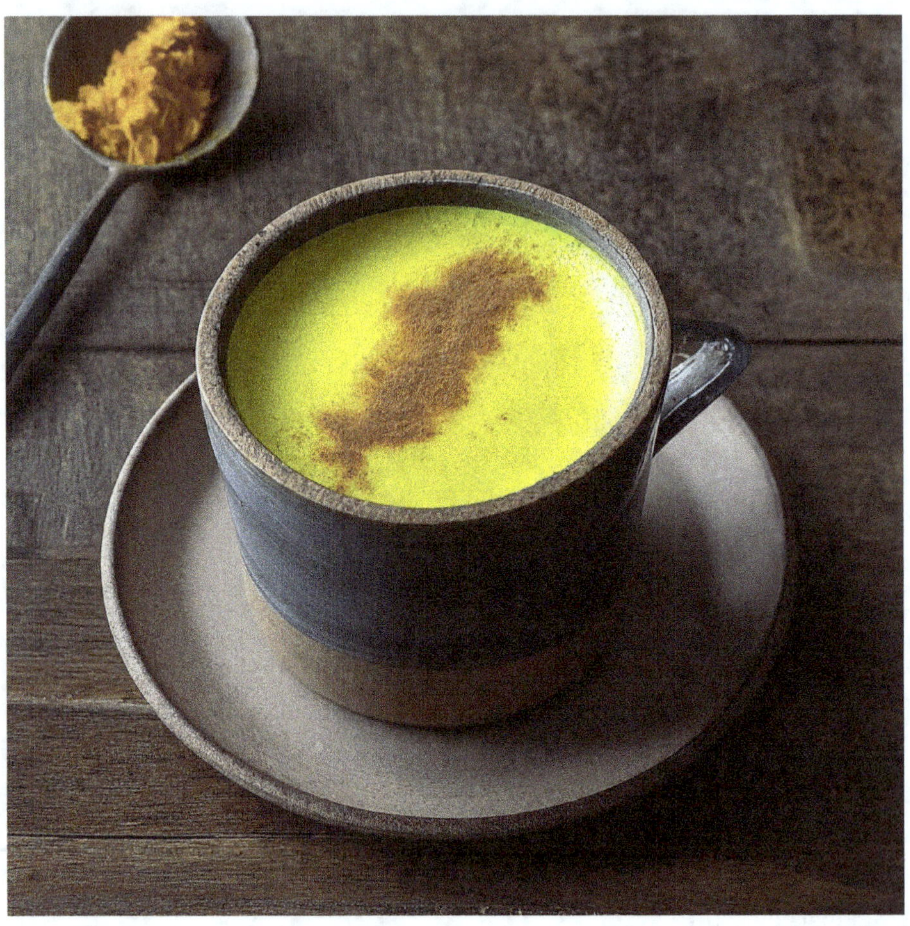

Turmeric Latte, also known as Golden Milk, is a warm and comforting beverage that's perfect for any time of the day. The combination of turmeric and spices provides a soothing and health-boosting drink.

Cooking Time: 10 minutes

Servings: 2

Ingredients:

- 2 cups unsweetened almond milk (or any low-histamine milk alternative)
- 1 teaspoon ground turmeric
- 1/2 teaspoon ground cinnamon
- 1/4 teaspoon ground ginger
- 1 tablespoon honey or maple syrup (if tolerated)
- 1/2 teaspoon vanilla extract
- Pinch of black pepper

Instructions:

1. In a small saucepan, combine the almond milk, turmeric, cinnamon, ginger, honey, vanilla extract, and black pepper.
2. Whisk the mixture over medium heat until it comes to a gentle simmer.
3. Reduce heat to low and simmer for 5 minutes, whisking occasionally.
4. Pour the turmeric latte into mugs and serve hot.

Tips:

- Adjust the sweetness to your taste preference.
- Use fresh ginger instead of ground ginger for a spicier kick.
- Garnish with a sprinkle of cinnamon on top.

Nutritional Info (per serving):

- Calories: 90
- Protein: 1g
- Carbohydrates: 18g
- Fat: 2g
- Fiber: 1g

* * *

Chamomile Tea

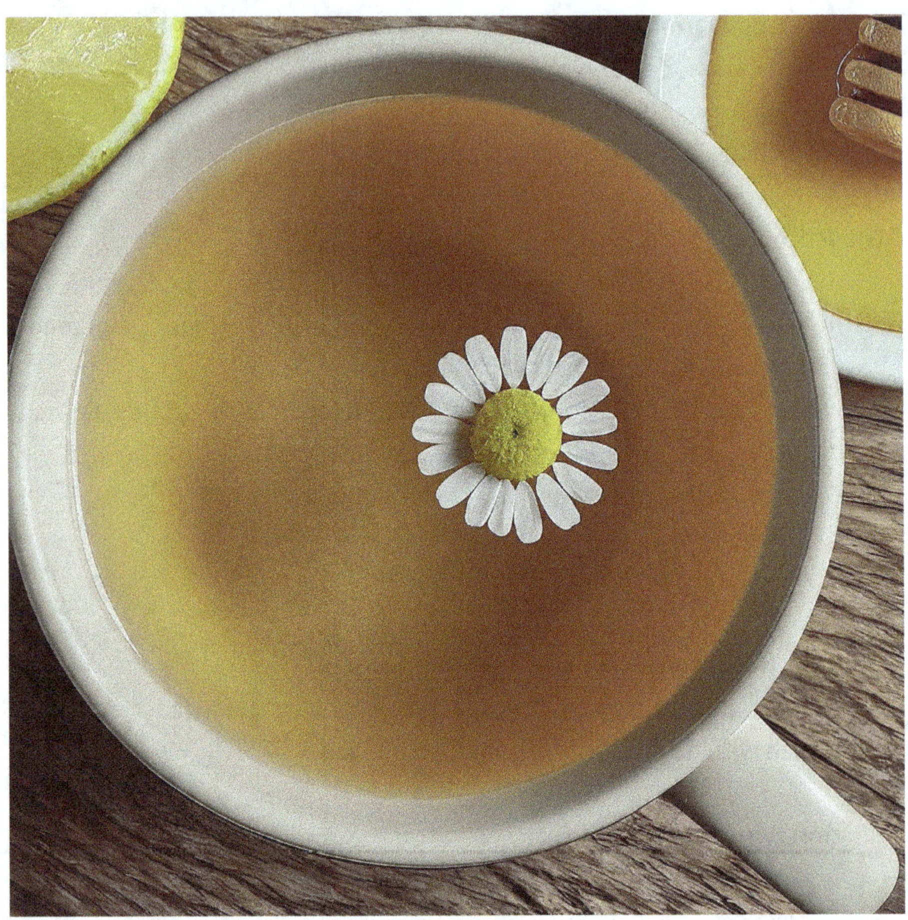

Chamomile Tea is a calming and soothing beverage that's perfect for unwinding. Known for its relaxing properties, chamomile tea can help promote better sleep and reduce stress.

Cooking Time: 10 minutes

Servings: 2

Ingredients:

- 2 cups water
- 2 chamomile tea bags or 2 tablespoons dried chamomile flowers
- Honey or lemon (optional, if tolerated)

Instructions:

1. Bring the water to a boil in a small saucepan.
2. Remove from heat and add the chamomile tea bags or dried chamomile flowers.
3. Let steep for 5–7 minutes.
4. Remove the tea bags or strain the tea to remove the flowers.
5. Pour the tea into mugs and add honey or lemon if desired.
6. Serve hot.

Tips:

- For a stronger flavor, steep the tea for a few extra minutes.
- Add a slice of fresh ginger or a cinnamon stick for additional flavor.
- Chamomile tea can also be enjoyed cold; simply refrigerate after steeping.

Nutritional Info (per serving):

- Calories: 2 (without honey or lemon)
- Protein: 0g
- Carbohydrates: 0g
- Fat: 0g
- Fiber: 0g

Meal Planning and Prep

Weekly Meal Planning Guide

1. Set Your Goals:

- Identify your dietary needs, preferences, and restrictions (e.g., low histamine, gluten-free).
- Consider your weekly schedule to determine when you have time to cook.

2. Plan Your Meals:

- Choose recipes for breakfast, lunch, dinner, and snacks that fit your dietary needs.
- Aim for a balance of protein, healthy fats, and complex carbohydrates in each meal.
- Plan for leftovers to save time and reduce food waste.

3. Make a Shopping List:

- Based on your meal plan, create a detailed shopping list.
- Organize the list by sections of the grocery store to streamline your shopping trip.
- Check your pantry and fridge before shopping to avoid buying duplicates.

4. Prep Ahead:

- Dedicate a few hours once or twice a week to meal prep.
- Wash and chop vegetables, cook grains, and portion out snacks to make weekday meals easier.

5. Stay Flexible:

- Be prepared to adjust your meal plan if necessary. Life happens, and flexibility is key.
- Keep a few quick and easy recipes on hand for busy days.

Tips for Batch Cooking

1. Choose Recipes Wisely:

- Select recipes that freeze well or can be easily reheated, such as soups, stews, casseroles, and grains.
- Avoid recipes that may become soggy or lose texture after reheating.

2. Invest in Quality Storage:

- Use airtight containers or freezer bags to store your batch-cooked meals.
- Label containers with the date and contents for easy identification.

3. Cook in Bulk:

- Double or triple recipes to ensure you have enough portions for multiple meals.
- Cook large batches of staple items like rice, quinoa, beans, and roasted vegetables.

4. Portion Control:

- Divide cooked meals into individual servings to make reheating quick and easy.
- Use portion control to avoid overeating and ensure balanced meals.

5. Cool and Store Properly:

- Allow hot foods to cool before refrigerating or freezing to prevent condensation and spoilage.
- Store meals in the refrigerator for up to 4 days or in the freezer for up to 3 months.

Sample Meal Plans

Sample Meal Plan 1:
Monday:

- Breakfast: Berry Banana Smoothie
- Lunch: Quinoa and Cucumber Salad
- Dinner: Baked Lemon Chicken with Roasted Vegetables
- Snack: Rice Cakes with Almond Butter

Tuesday:

- Breakfast: Overnight Oats with Coconut Milk
- Lunch: Mixed Greens with Pear and Walnut
- Dinner: Beef Stir-Fry with Fresh Vegetables
- Snack: Fresh Fruit Salad

Wednesday:

- Breakfast: Avocado Toast with Fresh Herbs
- Lunch: Turkey and Avocado Wrap
- Dinner: Grilled Salmon with Quinoa

- Snack: Coconut Macaroons

Thursday:

- Breakfast: Scrambled Eggs with Spinach
- Lunch: Lentil and Vegetable Stew
- Dinner: Chicken and Rice Casserole
- Snack: Hummus with Gluten-Free Crackers

Friday:

- Breakfast: Quinoa Breakfast Bowl with Fresh Berries
- Lunch: Carrot Ginger Soup
- Dinner: Zucchini Noodles with Pesto
- Snack: Guacamole with Veggie Sticks

Sample Meal Plan 2:
Monday:

- Breakfast: Turmeric Latte and Fresh Berry Parfait
- Lunch: Turkey and Avocado Wrap
- Dinner: Lentil and Vegetable Stew
- Snack: Coconut Macaroons

Tuesday:

- Breakfast: Avocado Toast with Fresh Herbs
- Lunch: Quinoa and Cucumber Salad
- Dinner: Baked Lemon Chicken with Roasted Vegetables
- Snack: Fresh Fruit Salad

Wednesday:

- Breakfast: Berry Banana Smoothie
- Lunch: Mixed Greens with Pear and Walnut
- Dinner: Beef Stir-Fry with Fresh Vegetables
- Snack: Hummus with Gluten-Free Crackers

Thursday:

- Breakfast: Scrambled Eggs with Spinach
- Lunch: Grilled Chicken Sandwich with Homemade Mayo
- Dinner: Grilled Salmon with Quinoa
- Snack: Rice Cakes with Almond Butter

Friday:

- Breakfast: Overnight Oats with Coconut Milk
- Lunch: Carrot Ginger Soup
- Dinner: Zucchini Noodles with Pesto
- Snack: Guacamole with Veggie Sticks

Budget-Friendly Meal Prep Ideas

1. Utilize Inexpensive Staples:

- Base meals around budget-friendly staples like rice, lentils, beans, oats, and seasonal vegetables.

2. Buy in Bulk:

- Purchase grains, beans, and spices in bulk to save money.
- Store bulk items properly to extend their shelf life.

3. Shop Seasonal and Local:

- Choose seasonal fruits and vegetables for better prices and freshness.
- Visit local farmers' markets for deals on fresh produce.

4. Plan for Leftovers:

- Cook larger portions and plan to use leftovers for lunches or dinners throughout the week.
- Repurpose leftovers into new meals, such as using roasted vegetables in a salad or stir-fry.

5. Freeze Extra Portions:

- Freeze portions of soups, stews, and casseroles for quick meals on busy days.
- Label and date freezer meals to keep track of what's available.

6. Make Your Own Snacks:

- Prepare homemade snacks like energy balls, granola bars, and fruit salads instead of buying pre-packaged items.
- Use inexpensive ingredients like oats, nuts, and dried fruit.

7. Batch Cook Breakfasts:

- Prepare large batches of breakfast items like overnight oats, chia pudding, and smoothie packs to save time and money.
- Store portions in the refrigerator or freezer for easy access.

By following this meal planning and prep guide, you can efficiently manage your time, stick to your dietary needs, and save money while enjoying delicious, low-histamine meals throughout the week.

Resources and References

List of Low Histamine Foods

Proteins:

- Freshly cooked chicken
- Freshly cooked turkey
- Freshly caught fish (e.g., cod, haddock, sole)
- Eggs
- Legumes (lentils, chickpeas, peas)

Fruits:

- Apples
- Pears
- Blueberries
- Strawberries
- Watermelon
- Mangos
- Cantaloupe

Vegetables:

- Carrots

- Zucchini
- Broccoli
- Kale
- Spinach (fresh)
- Sweet potatoes
- Cucumbers

Grains and Starches:

- Rice (white, brown, basmati)
- Quinoa
- Oats
- Buckwheat
- Millet

Dairy and Alternatives:

- Fresh milk (if tolerated)
- Plain yogurt (if tolerated)
- Coconut milk
- Almond milk
- Rice milk

Herbs and Spices:

- Basil
- Parsley
- Oregano
- Thyme
- Rosemary
- Ginger
- Turmeric

Oils and Fats:

- Olive oil
- Coconut oil
- Avocado oil

Others:

- Fresh herbs
- Homemade mayonnaise (using fresh ingredients)
- Coconut aminos (soy sauce alternative)

Helpful Websites and Books

Websites:

- **The Histamine Intolerance Awareness Site:** Provides detailed information on histamine intolerance, symptoms, and management. www.histamineintolerance.org.uk
- **Healing Histamine:** A comprehensive resource for recipes, research, and articles related to histamine intolerance. www.healinghistamine.com
- **Histamine Friendly Kitchen:** Offers a variety of low-histamine recipes and meal planning tips. www.histaminefriendlykitchen.com

Books:

- **"The Low Histamine Chef Cookbook" by Yasmina Ykelenstam:** This cookbook is filled with delicious and low-histamine recipes, along with tips for managing histamine intolerance.
- **"The Anti-Inflammatory Diet & Action Plans" by Dorothy Calimeris and Sondi Bruner:** Includes meal plans and recipes that are low in histamine and anti-inflammatory.
- **"Histamine Intolerance: A Comprehensive Guide for Healthcare Profes-

sionals" by Dr. Janice Joneja: An in-depth guide to understanding and managing histamine intolerance, suitable for both healthcare professionals and patients.

Support Groups and Forums

Online Support Groups:

- **Facebook Groups:**
- **Histamine Intolerance Support:** A community where members share tips, experiences, and support for managing histamine intolerance.
- **Low Histamine Chefs:** Focuses on sharing recipes and cooking tips for a low-histamine diet.
- **Reddit:**
- **r/HistamineIntolerance:** A subreddit where users discuss symptoms, treatments, and dietary strategies related to histamine intolerance.

Forums:

- **The Mastocytosis Society Forum:** Although focused on mastocytosis, this forum provides valuable information and support for those dealing with histamine-related issues. www.tmsforacure.org/forum
- **Histamine Intolerance Forum:** A dedicated forum for discussing all aspects of histamine intolerance, including symptoms, treatments, and recipes. www.histamineintolerance.net/forum

Local Support Groups:

- **Check with local health organizations or hospitals:** They often have information on support groups for dietary restrictions and food intolerances, including histamine intolerance.
- **Meetup.com:** Search for local groups focused on histamine intolerance or related dietary needs. www.meetup.com

These resources and references can provide valuable information, support, and community for managing histamine intolerance and maintaining a low-histamine diet. Use them to expand your knowledge, find new recipes, and connect with others who share similar experiences.

Conclusion

Embarking on a low-histamine diet can seem daunting at first, but remember that every step you take is a move towards better health and well-being. It's a journey of discovery, learning, and adapting, and you've already made a significant commitment to taking care of yourself by exploring this cookbook.

Final Tips for Staying on Track

1. Be Patient with Yourself:

- Transitioning to a low-histamine diet takes time. Be patient and kind to yourself as you learn which foods work best for you.
- It's okay to make mistakes or have setbacks. What's important is that you continue to move forward.

2. Stay Organized:

- Plan your meals and keep a well-stocked pantry of low-histamine staples to make cooking easier.
- Use meal planning tools and apps to help you stay organized and reduce stress.

3. Experiment and Enjoy:

- Don't be afraid to try new recipes and ingredients. Cooking should be an enjoyable and creative process.
- Explore different herbs and spices to keep your meals flavorful and exciting.

4. Listen to Your Body:

- Pay attention to how different foods make you feel. Keep a food diary to track symptoms and identify potential triggers.
- Adjust your diet as needed based on your body's responses.

5. Seek Support:

- Join support groups and forums to connect with others who are also managing histamine intolerance. Sharing experiences and tips can be incredibly helpful.
- Don't hesitate to consult with healthcare professionals or a dietitian who can provide personalized advice and support.

6. Focus on Freshness:

- Whenever possible, choose fresh, unprocessed foods. Fresh foods are typically lower in histamine and more nutritious.
- Prepare meals at home to have better control over ingredients and food quality.

7. Plan for Convenience:

- Prepare meals and snacks ahead of time to make staying on track easier, especially on busy days.
- Keep simple, low-histamine snacks on hand to prevent hunger and temptation to eat high-histamine foods.

8. Celebrate Your Successes:

- Acknowledge and celebrate your progress, no matter how small. Each positive change is a step towards better health.
- Treat yourself to your favorite low-histamine dishes and enjoy the journey.

Your dedication to managing histamine intolerance and improving your health through diet is truly commendable. This cookbook is designed to support you on this journey by providing delicious, budget-friendly, and easy-to-make recipes. As you continue to explore and enjoy these meals, you'll find that eating a low-histamine diet can be both satisfying and enjoyable.

Remember, you are not alone on this journey. There is a community of people who understand and share similar experiences. Reach out, share your successes and challenges, and continue to learn and grow. Here's to your health, happiness, and many delicious meals ahead!

About the Author

Lila Hayes is a passionate home cook and food enthusiast dedicated to creating delicious, nutritious, and budget-friendly recipes for those managing histamine intolerance. With a background in nutrition and a personal journey of navigating dietary restrictions, Lila understands the challenges and rewards of maintaining a specialized diet.

Driven by a love for food and a desire to help others, Lila has spent years researching and experimenting with low-histamine ingredients to develop recipes that are both satisfying and easy to prepare. Her goal is to make healthy eating accessible and enjoyable for everyone, regardless of dietary limitations.

When she's not in the kitchen, Lila enjoys spending time with her family, exploring farmer's markets, and connecting with others in the histamine intolerance community. Through her work, she hopes to inspire and empower individuals to take control of their health and enjoy the process of cooking and eating wholesome, flavorful meals.